COPING WITH ENDOMETRIOSIS

JO MEARS graduated from University College, London, in 1984 and then trained as a journalist at the London College of Printing. She worked for The Press Association, The *Daily Mirror* and *Me* magazine before becoming a freelance writer. She now regularly contributes health articles to national newspapers and magazines such as *Woman's Own* and *New Woman*.

Overcoming Common Problems Series

For a full list of titles please contact
Sheldon Press, Marylebone Road, London NW1 4DU

Overcoming Common Problems

COPING WITH
ENDOMETRIOSIS

Jo Mears

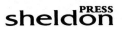

First published in Great Britain in 1996 by
Sheldon Press, SPCK, Marylebone Road, London NW1 4DU

Third impression 2001

British Library Cataloguing-in-Publication Data
A catalogue record for this book is available from the British Library

ISBN 0–85969–748–7

Photoset by Deltatype Ltd, Birkenhead, Merseyside
Printed in Great Britain by Biddles Ltd, *www.biddles.co.uk*

Acknowledgements

I would very much like to thank Diane Carlton, Kim Longlands, Dr B. I. Pirzada and Dr Michael Brush of the National Endometriosis Society for their help and support, as well as all the women suffering from endometriosis who kindly told me their stories.

Contents

Foreword

Endometriosis is a chronic and sometimes debilitating disease which can affect as many as 1 in 10 women from the onset of their periods to the menopause – and sometimes beyond.

Women with this perplexing disease often feel both pain and anger. Long delays in diagnosis cause women to doubt themselves and their symptoms, and the cyclical symptoms often cause others to doubt the sufferer too.

During my nurse-training in the late 1950s and early 1960s, there was only one paragraph on endometriosis in text-books. Since being diagnosed myself in 1980, and since I became involved with the National Endometriosis Society (NES) in 1981, I've seen the interest and information about endometriosis mushroom.

Women with endometriosis need simple, clear information to enable them to decide for themselves which kind of treatment may be right for them. This book is written in a clear question-and-answer format and covers everything from explanation, treatments and self-help. It is written by a sufferer for sufferers, and will fill a very important gap in the available information.

Our 1995 survey of 2,500 NES members showed that there is still an average delay of seven years in diagnosis, and an average loss of 45 working days per year per member. This makes an enormous impact on the lives of these women and on the economy of the country.

Women who are better informed will be able to gain earlier diagnosis and treatment, thus reducing the impact of this debilitating disease.

Jo Mears has worked closely with the NES in the writing of this book. We would like to thank her for writing a book aimed directly at women, in a language they can understand.

Diane Carlton
Chair to the NES Medical Advisory Panel

1

What is Endometriosis?

Some basic facts and figures

What does 'endometriosis' mean?

If you mention the word endometriosis to most people, they'll look at you blankly and say, 'Endo what?' But very occasionally you'll find someone who says, 'Oh yes. I've heard of that. My aunt has it. It's to do with painful periods isn't it?'

Painful periods are indeed one of the main symptoms of endometriosis, but the name itself is actually derived from the following Ancient Greek words:

- *end*, meaning inside
- *metra*, meaning womb
- *osis*, meaning disease, problem or abnormality.

What is endometriosis?

As its name suggests, endometriosis is an abnormality or problem connected with the womb. Endometriosis means that some of the tissue which lines the womb (endometrium) and is shed each month during a period, is found outside the womb. When anything in the body is found *outside* its normal site it is called 'ectopic'. So you may hear people say that endometriosis is caused by 'ectopic endometrium'.

How many women are affected?

- It is estimated that 10 per cent of women are affected, although some experts believe it could be as many as 20 per cent;
- it is the second most common gynaecological condition after fibroids.

Who is Affected?

Endometriosis most commonly affects women aged 25–40. But because it is linked to the monthly cycle it can occur at any time from when your period starts to when it stops (and in some women even continues afterwards). New research suggests that all women may have deposits of endometriosis but that, for reasons not yet fully understood, it only causes a problem in some women.

Why is it more common today?

Endometriosis was first discovered in 1860 by an Austrian doctor called von Rokitansky, but it wasn't named until 1924 when an American doctor, A. J. Sampson, described the condition and gave it the name of endometriosis.

That doesn't mean to say that endometriosis didn't exist before then! In fact, many endometriosis sufferers today believe their grandmothers may have suffered with the condition because they can remember them having very painful periods (one of the main symptoms), and because it's now believed that it may run in families to a certain extent.

However, as endometriosis usually regresses during pregnancy, it may have been less common in the past when most women spent a lot of their lives being pregnant. In our great-grandmothers' day, women usually only had about 35 periods during their lives, because they were so often pregnant, whereas these days the average woman has about 400 periods. Because endometriosis is associated with the menstrual bleed, it may be that the more periods you have, the more opportunity endometriosis has to develop.

Other reasons for the increase are:

- Doctors are better at diagnosing endometriosis because they are becoming more aware of the condition (although the situation is still far from perfect!).
- Doctors also have easier means of diagnosing it, through a laparoscopy – a telescopic, keyhole investigation whereby a doctor can actually see the endometriosis patches inside your body (see Chapter 4).
- Nowadays doctors also have ways of recognizing microscopic patches of endometriosis which might have been missed in the past and which can cause just as much trouble as larger, more visible areas.
- Women have more of a voice today and are less afraid of reporting their troublesome symptoms, which include painful intercourse.

Where do you get endometriosis?

The most common places for endometriosis to occur (see Figure 1) are:

- The **peritoneum** – the membrane-lining of the abdominal cavity – which is a kind of thin skin that goes round and protects all the organs, allowing them to move freely in the pelvis.
- On the surfaces of the **pelvic organs** such as the **ovaries** and **Fallopian tubes**.

Endometriosis: some facts and figures

The NES carried out a survey of sufferers in 1995. Here are a few of their findings:

- One woman in ten is thought to suffer from endometriosis.
- 57 per cent of sufferers were told, at some stage, that there was nothing wrong with them.
- On average, women with endometriosis symptoms wait three years before consulting their GP.
- 50 per cent of sufferers consulted their GP five times or more before obtaining a referral to a specialist.
- On average, it takes seven years from the first symptoms appearing to a woman receiving the correct diagnosis.
- Two-thirds of women in the survey had taken time off work because of the disease.
- The average time each woman lost from work each year was 45 days.

- Also on the surfaces of the **bowel** and **bladder** and on the **intestines** and in the **Pouch of Douglas** (a small flap and space behind the uterus, between the uterus and the rectum; endometriosis cells often settle here due to the pull of gravity, and doctors can often tell through an internal examination whether there is tenderness there – a sign that endometriosis is probably present).
- It has even been known to travel further afield to the lungs, nose, ears and even behind the eye – but this is far less common. In fact, it has been found just about everywhere in the body apart from the spleen (see Figure 1 for endometriosis hot-spots and occurrence rates).

What damage does endometriosis do?

Endometriosis hot-spots act like small patches of womb-lining and respond to the hormonal cycles which affect the womb. This means that these patches bleed during a monthly period – and as the blood has nowhere to go, it collects in the surrounding tissues.

This stray blood sometimes causes local irritation, leading to **inflammation** and **scarring** and can, in severe cases, produce **solid nodules** or **cysts** (such as the large chocolate cysts sometimes found on the ovaries – called chocolate because of their colour, caused by the dark blood collecting inside them).

This damage can also lead to the pelvic organs becoming stuck together

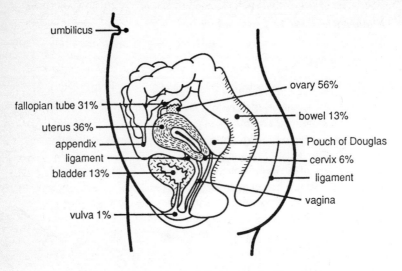

Figure 1: Endometriosis hot-spots in the pelvis
(percentages refer to the frequency at which sites are affected,
according to the 1984 NES survey).

which doctors refer to as **adhesions**. Adhesions are a web of scar-tissue resembling clingfilm which makes organs stick together and can cause intense pain during periods. These adhesions may also affect other pelvic areas such as the bowel, bladder, ovaries and Fallopian tubes – and damage to these may also affect a woman's fertility.

Some endometriosis spots can also be trapped inside the muscles of the womb wall (a condition called **adenomyosis**). These spots in the muscle wall can swell and cause more pain.

But to understand more about how endometriosis affects us, we need to understand a little more about how our bodies work.

How your body works

Let's first of all look at some of the different parts of the body which make up the reproductive organs.

On the outside

Vulva: the fleshy area around the openings of the vagina and the urethra (the tube leading from the bladder through which you wee).

Labia: flaps of skin, like lips, which form the entrance to the vagina.

Clitoris: the most sensitive spot, shielded by the inner folds, which swells during sexual arousal.

On the inside

Vagina: a sort of elastic, muscular tube which expands and contracts to make room for anything from a tampon, to a penis – or even a baby!

Cervix: the neck of the womb which protrudes into the vagina and which, when touched, feels a bit like the tip of the nose in some women.

Womb (also known as the **uterus**): although thick and muscular, it's normally just the size and shape of a pear, but expands during pregnancy. At the top, the womb branches out into the Fallopian tubes on either side. It usually tilts forwards towards the bladder, but in women with endometriosis it can tilt backwards (called 'retroverted' – see more about this in Chapter 2).

Ligaments: these are bands of strong tissue that keep the womb in place. They stretch across the pelvic cavity from the pelvic walls, the bladder and the rectum. The womb, the Fallopian tubes and the ovaries are all attached to these ligaments, but they should still be able to move easily around and not be firmly stuck in one place (as can often happen with endometriosis).

The Fallopian tubes: these curve outwards from the womb and down towards the ovaries. At their ends, they have finger-like projections called fimbriae which stretch towards the ovaries and catch the eggs when they are released from the ovaries. They're also lined with tiny, hair-like structures called cilia, which waft the egg down towards the womb.

Ovaries: About the size of a walnut, these are where the eggs, and the female sex-hormones oestrogen and progesterone, are made. We are born with eggs already in place, but their numbers drop to about 200,000–500,000 by puberty. Every month a number are stimulated to develop by hormones, but only one egg becomes fully developed and is released.

Egg follicles: these are the fluid-filled sacs or glands in the ovaries which contain thousands of immature cells which could grow into eggs if they are given the correct stimulus.

Facts about periods

- Periods start at an average age of 13.4 – but individually usually start between 10 and 16, although it can sometimes be earlier or later.
- The average age for stopping is 51, but again it can occur earlier or later.
- The average number of periods a year is 13.
- The menstrual cycle is normally assumed to be 28 days long – i.e. there are 28 days from the start of one period (called Day 1) until the start of the next one. However, in practice every woman varies, and a cycle could be anything from 21 to 35 days long, with variations on either side.
- A period can last from one to eight days, although three to five days is more usual.

How do your periods start?

The first period is the result of your ovaries being switched on by hormones produced by the pituitary gland (see below).

Where do hormones come from?

The hormones involved in the menstrual cycle come from three different places:

- The hypothalamus: part of the brain just above the pituitary which controls the body's hormone activity, including stimulation of the pituitary gland in the menstrual cycle.
- The pituitary gland: a pea-sized organ at the base of the skull which produces a hormone that switches on the ovaries (among other things).
- The ovaries: the place where the eggs are produced.

What do hormones do?

A hormone is a chemical which sends messages to different parts of our body telling them to act in a certain way. Our periods are controlled and regulated by several different hormones, which are produced by the parts of the body mentioned above.

What happens during the menstrual cycle?

For the purposes of this explanation, we will assume that the menstrual cycle lasts 28 days. Day 1 is the first day of a period and Day 28 the last period-free day before bleeding starts again.

The menstrual phase (Days 1–5)

1 The hypothalamus produces a hormone called gonadotrophin-releasing hormone (GnRH) which stimulates the pituitary gland.
2 The pituitary in turn is stimulated into producing a hormone called follicle stimulating hormone (FSH).
3 FSH acts on the egg follicles, stimulating them into ripening and producing the female hormone called **oestrogen**.

The follicular phase (Days 6–12)

1 Oestrogen-levels in the blood then rise and are carried in the bloodstream to the womb where they cause the womb to start thickening.
2 FSH stops when the womb is thick enough and another hormone, LH (luteinizing hormone), starts to be released.
3 LH then triggers the ovulatory phase.

The ovulatory phase (Days 13–15)

1 LH causes one of the maturing follicles to burst and release an egg. Some women feel pain at this time – which doctors call Mittelschmerz, meaning literally 'pain in the middle'.
2 By this time, the open ends of the Fallopian tubes have moved closer to the ovaries making them ready to catch the released egg.
3 The cilia hairs which line the Fallopian tubes waft the egg down one of the tubes and into the womb. (At this time the vaginal mucus is thin to enable sperm to swim easily.)

The luteal phase (Days 16–23)

By the time the egg has wafted down the tube, this phase has already begun.

1 After the collapse of the egg follicle, cells proliferate and form a yellow cyst called the corpus luteum (meaning 'yellow body'). The corpus luteum then begins its own hormone production, starting to manufacture another female hormone called **progesterone**.
2 Progesterone stops any more follicles ripening, and helps to develop the womb even further, making it soft and spongy and secreting food for when the egg arrives.
3 The womb continues to thicken as the egg spends a further seven to eight days travelling down to the womb. If you are to become pregnant, the egg must meet live sperm in the first 12–24 hours after the egg is released and

before it begins to decay. (Vaginal mucus is thick at this time to prevent more sperm coming in.)

4 If the egg is fertilized by a sperm, it in turn secretes another hormone into the bloodstream called HCG (human chorionic gonadotrophin), which stimulates the corpus luteum to go on making progesterone, which in turn makes the womb develop even further. (Progesterone production is eventually taken over by the placenta and continues throughout pregnancy to stop the womb being shed.)

5 However, if the egg is *not* fertilized, no HCG is produced, the corpus luteum breaks down after seven days, and progesterone production stops.

The premenstrual phase (Days 24–28)

1 Now oestrogen and progesterone levels fall sharply.

2 During the following seven days, in response to the drop in progesterone-levels, the muscles in the womb-walls spasm and cut off the blood supply to the womb causing the lining to break down and be expelled as a period. Usually two-thirds of the womb-lining is shed, while the remaining one-third – a basic, deep layer – remains.

3 At the end of a period, progesterone and oestrogen levels are at their lowest in the blood, which triggers the production of GnRH again, then FSH and LH, and so the whole cycle starts again!

What goes wrong in women with endometriosis?

When the womb responds to hormonal changes and goes into spasm, as well as forcing some of the menstrual fluid down out of the cervix it also forces some out of the top of the womb through the Fallopian tubes and into the pelvic area. This process is called **retrograde menstruation**, and is thought by many to be the cause of endometriosis (see Chapter 2).

What is menstrual 'blood'?

The top two-thirds of the womb-lining (the endometrium) is shed during a period: it includes red blood cells, mucus, hormones, hormone-like structures called prostaglandins, tissue debris, and so on. But our main interest is in the live endometrial cells from the womb-lining which are thought possibly to attach themselves (via retrograde menstruation) to other areas in the pelvis, and which then begin to grow.

What is endometrial tissue?

Endometrial tissue is womb-lining which can cause a problem when it is found outside the womb. It appears in lots of different forms: as we discussed earlier, it can form as microscopic patches, cysts, nodules, and so on. Whatever form the endometriosis takes, the tissue it produces is made up of cells similar to the lining of the womb. They are often referred to by different names (as listed below) but basically they are all the same thing:

- **endometrial** tissue, patches, deposits, spots or implants;
- **endometriotic** blisters, lesions, vesicles or cells.

Is endometriosis life-threatening?

One of the biggest worries when women are first diagnosed with endometriosis is whether the condition is life-threatening in any way. Women with endometriosis could in theory die from related complications – such as septicaemia resulting from an obstructed bowel – but it isn't likely, and fortunately there is no known case of a woman dying directly as a result of endometriosis. The major problem with endometriosis is that it's a chronic condition (i.e. of slow duration, involving very slow changes), as well as being very painful and debilitating.

2

What causes endometriosis?

No one knows for sure what causes endometriosis. What is known, though, from tests on endometrial cells found outside the womb, is that they are similar to those lining the womb. But just how they got there isn't really clear.

Some researchers believe that women with endometriosis are born with endometrial deposits in places other than the womb, while others think these cells somehow move there from the womb in later life.

There are many more theories besides these, but no single theory has been wholly proved and it is highly likely that endometriosis could be the result of a combination of some of them. Here are some of the theories in bit more detail.

Retrograde menstruation

The most popular and oldest theory is that endometriosis is caused by retrograde menstruation (when some of the menstrual blood flows backwards in the wrong direction). Muscle-spasms during a period are thought sometimes to force the menstrual blood backwards up the Fallopian tubes and out into the pelvic cavity.

To understand this theory you need to remember the nature of your reproductive organs. As you might recall from the diagram in Chapter 1, the vagina leads up to the cervix which then leads into the womb. The top of the womb then branches out into the Fallopian tubes on either side, which are directed towards the ovaries. In many diagrams, the Fallopian tubes seem to join up with the ovary – but in fact there is a gap between them. When an egg is released from the ovaries each month, it doesn't fall down this gap because it is protected by the small finger-like projections (fimbriae) which direct the egg into the Fallopian tubes.

But when menstrual blood is forced back up the Fallopian tubes by muscle spasms during a period, it *does* slip down this gap into the pelvic cavity. This theory is backed up by research which shows that some of this stray menstrual blood contains active cells from the lining of the womb (which are then thought to implant elsewhere in the pelvic cavity).

There follows a brief summary of some of the experiments which support this theory.

- A lot of endometriosis is found in the lower part of the pelvis – which is the obvious place for the stray blood to collect. Also, a lot of endometrial deposits are found near the ends of the Fallopian tubes, which are the closest sites to the gap.
- In experiments, endometrial cells have been planted in the peritoneal cavity (the membrane of the abdominal cavity) and have taken root and grown.
- Live endometrial cells have been found in menstrual blood, and in the Fallopian tubes and peritoneal fluid.
- The female hormones oestrogen and progesterone have been found to be important for the long-term survival of endometrial implants.
- Women with a tight or closed-off cervical canal appear to be more likely to get endometriosis – in other words, the build-up of pressure in the womb could cause menstrual blood to flow backwards.
- Most women having periods have been found to have a certain amount of retrograde menstruation. In one study of women having keyhole surgery during their period, 90 per cent of those with normal Fallopian tubes were found to have quite a lot of blood in their peritoneal cavity.

The question is, why do stray endometrial cells in menstrual blood take root in some women and not in others? If you read on, the auto-immune system theory may go some way to explaining this.

Other theories

Auto-immune theory

This is another popular theory. Many scientists believe the immune system plays a key role in endometriosis. It's thought that a healthy immune system usually prevents normal body cells from implanting in unusual sites. Stray endometrial cells found in the pelvic cavity would usually be eaten up or destroyed by the body's own natural defences, and so wouldn't be able to implant. However, for some reason this system either doesn't work or over-reacts in endometriosis sufferers. They also think this alteration in the immune system might be passed on from generation to generation.

Bloodstream theory

Some researchers believe that live endometrial cells somehow pass into the bloodstream during a period and travel around body. They say this accounts for the fact that endometriosis is sometimes found in unusual sites which have a rich blood supply – such as the lungs or body muscles.

Lymphatic theory

This theory suggests that live endometrial cells somehow pass into the lymphatic system during a period. The lymphatic system is a complete system of vessels (like blood vessels) which carry nutrients to and from tissues and which also help to keep the immune system working. Some scientists say that this explains why endometriosis is sometimes found in lymphatic areas such as around the navel, which is rich in lymphatic vessels draining the pelvic area.

Waste ova theory

This theory suggests that some of the eggs which are released every month slip down in the gap between the Fallopian tubes and ovaries, and that some of cells attached to the egg develop into endometriosis sites under certain hormonal conditions.

Embryonic cell rests theory

This is a theory that some female embryos develop duplicate Mullerian Ducts (the structures in an embryo which eventually develop into adult reproductive organs). These Mullerian cells, which are known as 'rests', then develop into patches of functioning endometrium in later life.

Coelomic metaplasia theory

Metaplasia means the changing of one type of cell into another. This theory suggests that patches of endometrial cells are formed before birth in other places besides the womb, and that they lie dormant in some women but are somehow activated in endometriosis sufferers. Alternatively, normal cells are thought to change suddenly into endometrial cells, triggered perhaps by contact with stray endometrial cells.

Surgical causes

Certain types of surgery – such as having a Caesarean, a D & C, a hysterectomy or treatment for fibroids – have been linked to triggering endometriosis because they stir up the bottom lining of the womb, which could make it implant elsewhere.

Dioxins

One new school of thought has looked into the possibility that man-made chemicals called dioxins may be a cause of endometriosis. They believe that dioxins may behave like hormones, causing oestrogen-levels to rise. Dioxins are by-products of manufacturing processes involving chlorine – such as plastic, PVC, solvents, pesticides, wood preservatives, disinfectants and drugs. They are produced when the waste containing these

Possible thyroid link

One researcher, Dr Michael Brush, believes that some women with endometriosis may be suffering from a thyroid dysfunction. In a survey of the thyroid function and endocrine levels (hormones secreted from glands like the pituitary) of 120 women with endometriosis, he found that, although their routine thyroid tests were normal, the incidence of thyroid auto-antibodies was 20 per cent higher than the reported percentage incidence in other women. In some cases, the levels of thyroid auto-antibodies were consistent with a definite thyroid auto-immune disease. Some of these cases were treated by GPs with low-dose thyroxine and the women's health improved considerably.

chlorines is burnt. They then go into the air and fall on to the grass and plants, where they are then eaten by animals such as cows. Animal fats, such as meat and diary produce, are thought to be the major source of dioxins in humans.

Research in America suggests that dioxins attack the immune system causing problems such as low sperm-counts and a high incidence of endometriosis in women.

Researchers at the Women's Environmental Health Network (see Useful Addresses at the back of the book) even estimate that dioxins could affect between one and eight per cent of unborn babies, and are looking to see how this might affect their fertility in later life. It is also thought that dioxins could lead to change in thyroid function and immune system.

Heredity: does endometriosis run in families?

Endometriosis does seem to be hereditary. If a close relative (i.e. a mother, sister or aunt) suffers from endometriosis, you are 7–10 per cent more likely to suffer from it yourself. However, scientists are not yet sure whether this is due to an inherited gene or environmental factors which are 'inherited' from our relatives – such as a tendency to smoke or eat a certain type of diet. It's also been discovered that women with a very close relative suffering from endometriosis are more likely to get it severely, and that it seems to be passed on through the mother's family.

Other possible causes

Delayed motherhood

Pregnancy is known to protect against endometriosis because, during pregnancy, you don't have periods and so there is less chance of retrograde menstruation. It is also thought that the high levels of oestrogen and progesterone in the body during pregnancy may somehow protect against endometriosis.

But just because you delay motherhood doesn't mean that you will definitely suffer from endometriosis. Delayed motherhood can, however, sometimes be the result of endometriosis: some women with endometriosis do take longer to get pregnant (see Chapter 8).

A 'career-woman's disease'

Doctors often used to refer to endometriosis as the career-woman's disease, because career-women who often delayed motherhood were more frequently reported to be suffering from endometriosis. However, this is now thought to be incorrect, as the early studies didn't take into account such things as attitudes to period pain or willingness to question a diagnosis (in other words, career-women might be better able to complain, but it doesn't mean that other types of women aren't suffering, too). Indeed, endometriosis has now been found to affect all sectors of society including teenagers, ethnic minority groups and even women after the menopause. (The 1995 survey revealed that diagnosis may be delayed in some cases by the belief that endometriosis is an older woman's disease – whereas two-thirds of respondents had noticed some symptoms before the age of 25.)

> Jacqueline, 34, who was diagnosed as having endometriosis and fibroids says: 'I think there was a delay in my diagnosis because I'm black and I kept getting sent off to the sexually transmitted diseases clinic – even though I'd only ever had two boyfriends. Then, when I was eventually diagnosed after undergoing a laparoscopy, the doctor looked at me quizzically and said, ''That's strange – you seem too young to get endometriosis''. Having read more about it since, I realize it can affect just about any woman of any age!'

The position of the womb

In most women, the womb tilts slightly forwards and the cervix points slightly backwards. But in some women, the womb may be tilted further forward (anteverted), or be tilted backwards (retroverted) with the cervix pointing forwards.

Some studies suggest that women with a womb which tilts backwards may be twice as likely to get endometriosis; but other experts dispute this. The reason for this isn't known – although it may be that this position makes it easier for cells in retrograde menstruation to settle in the pelvis.

Endometriosis can in fact cause problems in women with all types of uterus. However, women who have a retroverted or anteverted uterus may have the added problem of the uterus being fixed in a rigid position because of surrounding adhesions (see Chapter 1 for an explanation of adhesions).

The IUD & Pill

Some women feel they have made themselves vulnerable to endometriosis because they have been on the Pill which affects hormones – and we know that hormones play a big role in endometriosis.

Early versions of the Pill contained relatively large amounts of oestrogen, and this could have made women more susceptible by increasing the amount of endometrium-stimulating oestrogen in the body; but more recent ones, containing high levels of progesterone, are thought to protect against endometriosis. This is because progesterone is the hormone responsible for breaking down the womb and which generally also has the effect of softening and breaking down endometrial deposits.

There are similar worries about the IUD which, to a certain extent, works as a contraceptive by irritating the womb lining. But this has not so far been found to increase the risk of endometriosis.

Tampons

Some women fear that tampons may cause retrograde menstruation by blocking the exit of blood from womb. Again, there is no evidence of this – although teenage girls with obstructions (such as a narrow cervix) have been found to be much more likely to develop endometriosis. If you are worried you could use sanitary towels more often or perhaps just during the night.

Maria, 32, who suffers from endometriosis in the bladder area says: 'I find that tampons seem to make my period pain worse and sometimes are even impossible to insert. I'm much happier using sanitary towels and only sometimes use tampons at the end of my period.'

Stress

Obviously suffering pain a lot of the time does lead to stress, and stress is now known to depress the immune system, dampening down the action of the white blood-cells which help destroy invading organisms. As yet, the role of stress and the auto-immune dysfunction in endometriosis isn't fully understood, but it is an area of continuing research.

3

Have I got endometriosis?

What are the symptoms?

Pain is the most common symptom of endometriosis and the reason most sufferers go to their doctor (94% of sufferers in the 1984 National Endometriosis Society survey reported pain). However, the extent of the pain doesn't seem to be dependent on how much endometriosis you have but rather *where* it is. For instance, a small number of cysts in an area which is disturbed during intercourse may be much more painful than a larger number elsewhere. Most sufferers also report that their pain seems to get worse during their period, although many other sufferers also report experiencing constant pain. Generally, however, if the pain comes and goes during your menstrual cycle, it's highly suggestive of endometriosis.

There are five classic symptoms of endometriosis (the percentages refer to the number of sufferers in the 1984 survey who experienced the symptom):

- painful periods (known as dysmenorrhoea) – 94%;
- painful intercourse (dyspareunia) – 55%;
- pelvic pain, including painful bowel movements – 48% and constipation – 45%;
- infertility – 41%;
- painful urination – 26%.

Some of the other commonly reported symptoms are:

- painful ovulation;
- heavy periods, including loss of blood-clots and stale brown blood;
- abnormal bleeding;
- depression;
- premenstrual syndrome;
- back-pain.

Painful periods

Many women complain of painful cramps which often reach their peak two days after their period has started. But how do you know whether your periods are more painful than anyone else's? It is particularly hard to tell, as we are all brought up to think that it's normal for periods to be painful.

16

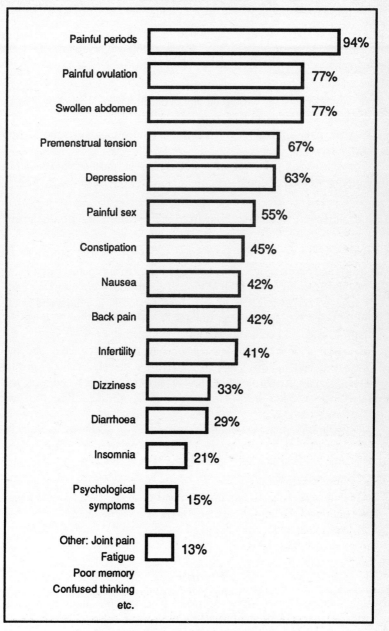

Figure 2: The symptoms of endometriosis
(percentages indicate the proportion of sufferers affected,
according to the 1984 NES survey).

Are your periods painful?

The following questions may help you to decide whether your period pain is severe. The more you answer 'Yes', the more likely you are to suffer from period pain which may be caused by endometriosis.

1 Do you take days off work each month because of menstrual cramps, or wake up at night because of them?
2 Is your pain so bad that it can't be relieved by over-the-counter painkillers?
3 Are your period pains getting worse each year, or does your pain last longer with each period?

This is how some women suffering from endometriosis describe their pain.

Jenny, a 40-year-old women's refuge worker diagnosed with endometriosis and fibroids, says: 'The first time I went to my doctor complaining about my period pains, I felt as though my insides were dropping out. I explained that I was often off work for three weeks at a time, and would be crippled by the pain and running a high temperature. During my period, often all I could do was just lie in the bath crying.'

Linda, a 28-year-old kitchen planner who discovered she had extensive endometriosis which included the bowel, recalls: 'I always have a gripping pain shooting right through my stomach and back, and feel very sick and dizzy. Every month I have to take time off work because of it.'

Lynn, a 38-year-old building society worker, diagnosed with endometriosis and an ovarian cyst, says, 'The pain during my period was so bad that I couldn't go out, and the painkillers the doctor kept prescribing were absolutely useless.'

Take note: two-thirds of respondents in the 1995 survey had taken time off work because of endometriosis.

Painful sex

Painful intercourse is often a main indicator of endometriosis, as intercourse can disturb endometrial patches or scar-tissue in the pelvic area. But understandably many women are reluctant to mention this symptom to their doctors – and this can often delay a diagnosis (more on this in Chapter 4).

Do you have painful sex?

You should seek help if you experience any of the following:

1 You are avoiding sex because it hurts during or after sex.
2 You feel a deep pain in your vagina during intercourse.
3 Sex is more painful at certain times of the month or in specific positions.

Jenny says: 'My husband and I hadn't had sex for a year-and-a-half before I finally went to see a gynaecologist. If we tried to have sex, it would not only hurt at that immediate time but the pain would go on for days afterwards.'

Lesley, a 29-year-old care worker, says: 'Sex in certain positions was excruciatingly painful. For me, one night of active sex meant two weeks of pain afterwards.'

Jackie, a 33-year-old science administrator who suffers from severe endometriosis, says: 'Sex for me is like making love to a bayonet. I get pain during and after intercourse, and even pain with the big ''O'' if I ever get that far! Sometimes I also bleed afterwards. I couldn't understand why it was so painful until, after a laser laparoscopy, a deeply embedded nodule was found at the top of the vagina, in the wall of tissue between the vagina and the rectum. I was extremely annoyed because the gynaecologist had previously said to me, ''Some women will experience painful intercourse and the reasons aren't always physical'', which had meant I'd gone on suffering with pain for nine months before the real reason was discovered.'

Pelvic pain

Pelvic pain is basically pain in the pelvic area. The pelvis is the bony structure in the lower abdomen, formed by the hip-bones, sacrum and coccyx, which protects organs such as the bowel, bladder and ovaries. Pain in this area might occur mid-cycle when you ovulate and your eggs are released (also known as Mittelschmerz).

Vanessa, a 24-year-old beauty therapist, suffered mid-cycle pain: 'I found that the pain when I was ovulating was the worst,' she says. 'It was an excruciating pain all down the right side of my abdomen. Once it got so bad I collapsed and had to be rushed to hospital. It was the sort of pain which nothing could blot out.'

Pelvic pain can also occur before, during and after your period (see Figure 3). Some women even complain of experiencing a dull pain in the pelvic area all the time.

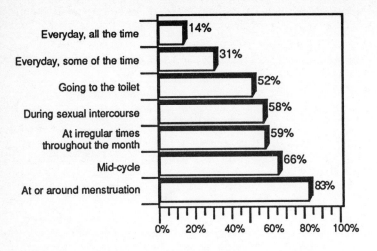

Figure 3: When pain occurs – the proportion of sufferers
who experience pain at different times
(according to the 1993 NES survey).

Paula, a 36-year-old mother-of-two, diagnosed with endometriosis on the ovary and womb ligaments, says: 'In my early twenties I found I was getting pain all the time, which meant I had to take a lot of time off work. If I hadn't been working for such a sympathetic employer I'm sure I would have been sacked.'

Grace, a 29-year-old student who's been treated for fibroids and severe endometriosis, comments: 'I've had very painful periods ever since I was ten. The pain was excruciating, and by the time I was in my twenties I was experiencing pain for two weeks every month. It was a sort of constant nag, and my abdomen always felt sore. I also felt a sharp pain whenever I sat down, and if I walked it would get worse.'

But sometimes this sort of pain can be caused by other conditions which may have to be ruled out first (see the end of the chapter).

Do you have pelvic pain?

The following questions might help. Again, the more times you answer 'Yes', the more likely you are to suffer from pelvic pain caused by endometriosis.

1 Do certain movements or positions – such as walking, running, sitting or lying down – cause you pelvic pain?
2 Do you have low back-pain before, during or after your period?
3 Does a bowel movement or urination become painful during your period?

Kim, 36, married with one daughter and diagnosed with moderate endometriosis behind the womb, says: 'Ever since I was a teenager I've had terrible periods which have involved constipation and diarrhoea. I'd often get constipation for up to ten days before my period started, and would spend hours on the loo, with my mum having to pass me magazines to read while I was sitting there! Then, once my period started, I'd get diarrhoea. My doctor just put it down to me being a neurotic teenager!'

Linda says: 'I'd usually get diarrhoea leading up to my period and then constipation for three to four days afterwards. I also had horrible cystitis-like symptoms during my period, and the pain was almost unbearable when I went to the loo. My doctor kept diagnosing a fibre problem. But once, when he wasn't there, I saw a locum who sent me for a scan and later a laparoscopy which revealed a cyst on my ovary, endometriosis on most of my pelvic organs and bladder, with possible bowel complications which are still being investigated.'

Judith, a 53-year-old farmer and counsellor, says, 'I'd never had any problems with periods when suddenly one night I had to get up and go to the loo at least three times. I got something from the chemist for cystitis, but it didn't help at all. It just got worse and worse. The GP eventually diagnosed a urine infection and put me on an antibiotic called Septrin. I was then sent to see a urologist and underwent a cystoscopy (a type of bladder examination) and kidney X-rays. When these revealed nothing, I was finally sent to a gynaecologist. He suggested endometriosis and put me on danazol; eventually I had a laparoscopy which revealed endometrial scarring around the bladder area.'

Infertility

Between 30 and 50 per cent of women investigated for infertility are found to be suffering from endometriosis. However, it's still not clear whether endometriosis causes infertility, whether it's just somehow associated with it, or if it is simply a coincidental finding. The following questions might help you to decide whether your infertility could be associated with endometriosis – but for more information on infertility see Chapter 8.

Could you be suffering from infertility?

1 Have you been trying unsuccessfully to get pregnant for more than a year?
2 Have you been having sex just during your fertile periods but still haven't fallen pregnant?
3 Have you experienced more than one miscarriage?

Helen, a 35-year-old accountant, says, 'Since I'd started my periods they were so painful that I'd often pass out. But it was only when I read an article about painful periods that I wondered whether endometriosis might be the cause. The slight suspicion that I might have endometriosis deepened in my thirties when I tried for two years to get pregnant, without success. I was then advised to have a laparoscopy and mild endo was diagnosed. But they also said I had a kink in one of my Fallopian tubes and that one of my ovaries was quite far from Fallopian tube. I went on drug treatment followed by IVF, but eventually fell pregnant naturally.'

Other symptoms

Heavy periods

Officially a heavy period is said to occur when over 80 ml of blood is lost – but we are hardly likely to get out a measuring jug to see if we fall into this category. However, the following are indicators of a heavy period:

- frequent flooding – when your tampon or sanitary towel is unable to hold the flow and needs to be changed constantly (i.e. two hourly);
- your menstrual flow includes blood clots (usually blood clots are broken down by a specific enzyme, but when there's a lot of blood it can't cope and so clots appear);
- you are suffering from anaemia (which can be due to heavy blood loss).

Kim recalls: 'During my period, blood would come out as I sat on the toilet as though I was passing urine. I had to change my sanitary towel every hour, and I would always have to change my sheets because I leaked in bed at night.'

Abnormal bleeding

The following are types of abnormal bleeding which can occur as a result of endometriosis:

- irregular periods;

22

- having your periods more often, i.e. your cycle gets progressively shorter;
- spotting before your period, or bleeding mid-cycle;
- dark discharge following your period.

Grace says: 'In my twenties, my cycle seemed to get shorter and shorter, going down from every 29 days to every 23. And most of the time I felt nauseous and in pain.'

Whereas Fiona, a 28-year-old office manager, says: 'After I came off the Pill in my early twenties I had horrendous periods which lasted for eight to ten days. They were so bad I couldn't eat a thing, and I lost a lot of weight.'

Depression

Quite high levels of depression are reported by endometriosis sufferers – often because pain can be very hard to cope with. It can make you feel tense and irritable and lead to feeling run-down, depressed and lacking in self-esteem. This in turn can lower your pain threshold. Worries about infertility can also add to this; and the confusion and lack of understanding about endometriosis may make you feel that you have no control over the illness. Chapter 9 deals with some of the ways in which you can break this vicious circle. But in the meantime it may just help to realize that it's a normal reaction, and not to blame yourself for feeling the way you do.

PMS

Endometriosis is thought to be one of the triggers of premenstrual syndrome (PMS) – the name now given to the troublesome symptoms we often feel just before a period. There are 150 symptoms now listed, but some of the most common ones are mood changes, bloating, weight-gain, depression and food cravings.

Irene, a 40-year-old market research assistant, says: 'At least ten days before my period I'd get terrible mood-swings and tiredness. I felt I couldn't cope, and if I just knocked a cup of tea over I'd feel like jumping out of the window. I became fanatical about cleaning, and would snap at everyone and pick on my daughter. Also I slept very badly, and had quite a sore chest – bad enough for me not to be able to put my seat belt on. As soon as my period started, these feelings would lift. When eventually I began to get awful pain down my right side and PMS symptoms at other times of the month, I decided to have a hysterectomy. During the operation the ovaries were found to be riddled with endometriosis.'

Back Pain

Constant lower back-pain is reported by 42% of endometriosis sufferers, while 37% only experience it during their periods. In some cases the pain could be due to endometrial deposits around the intestines (i.e. stomach and bowel areas).

> Lesley says: 'Six months after having laser treatment for an abnormal cervical smear, I began to experience low back-pain continually, which became worse on getting out of bed in the morning. I didn't think this pain was cyclical because I had it all the time, and it began to drive me mad.'

Conditions which are confused with endometriosis

One problem with diagnosing endometriosis is that it can easily be confused with other conditions, such as those described below.

Pelvic inflammatory disease (PID): As its name suggests, this is an inflammation of the pelvis usually involving the uterus, Fallopian tubes and ovaries. Because it can cause painful sex, nagging pain and heavy periods, it's often considered as the first explanation for these symptoms, especially if you have a history of PID.

Fibroids: These are benign tumours of fibrous or muscular tissue which develop in the wall of the womb and which can cause heavy bleeding and similar symptoms to PID.

Kidney stones: These are calcified deposits in the kidneys which can cause intermittent, sharp pain or a constant dull ache.

Cystitis: This, and other urinary tract infections, are often confused with endometriosis. Cystitis is basically an infection caught when bacteria from the rectum get into the urethra, making you want to pass water frequently (and painfully).

Ectopic pregnancy: This is where the foetus develops in Fallopian tubes, often because they are blocked or inflamed. It often results in a sudden pain in the stomach area radiating up to the collar-bone.

Crohn's Disease: A condition in which segments of the alimentary tract become inflamed, thickened and ulcerated.

Irritable bowel syndrome (IBS): This causes recurrent abdominal pain with constipation or diarrhoea and is thought to be stress-induced. (The 1995 survey showed that 18 per cent of endometriosis sufferers were inappropriately referred to a gastroenterologist, 40% of whom were incorrectly diagnosed as having either IBS or Crohn's Disease.)

Salpingitis: This is an inflammation of one or both of the Fallopian tubes caused by bacterial infection spreading from the vagina, womb or blood, usually causing a sharp pain in the lower abdomen.

Take Note!

Because the symptoms of endometriosis can be caused by some of these other conditions, you should seek a doctor's help immediately if you experience any of them. However, once these other conditions have been ruled out, endometriosis should be suspected – especially if your symptoms are cyclical and only seem to occur leading up to or during your period.

'I was misdiagnosed for 18 years'

Jenny says: 'It took me 18 years to get a proper diagnosis. I got my first symptoms at 22 – symptoms such as a dull ache behind the navel, painful periods and sex. The doctor was very unsympathetic; at first he suggested it could be a sexually transmitted disease. Then, over the years, he diagnosed salpingitis, cystitis, a kidney infection and irritable bowel syndrome. In the end it was a female friend who listened to my symptoms and suggested endometriosis, and I demanded to see a consultant who discovered I had endometriosis and two fibroids!'

Lesley recalls: 'The first time I went to the doctor complaining of low back-pain and pain after sex, he said it was an infection and put me on a week-long course of antibiotics. When the antibiotics didn't help, he just kept on prescribing me different courses of antibiotics. Then PID was diagnosed (in spite of negative vaginal swabs!) and a water infection (in spite of a urine sample again being clear of infection). Then it was irritable bowel syndrome and a suspected ovarian cyst. It was only when I read an article about endometriosis that alarm bells started to ring, and I demanded that my GP send me for a laparoscopy. Mild endometriosis was finally diagnosed. I was so relieved that they had found something and my pain was now being taken seriously. I've since found out that I was actually lucky, because the average delay in diagnosis is about seven years.'

Other endometriosis terms

You may hear the following terms being used in connection with endometriosis:

Endometrioma: an endometrial cyst on the ovary.

Adenomyosis: when endometrial glands grow in the wall of the womb.

Ovarian cyst: a fluid-filled sac which develops on the ovary. If cysts become large and twist on their stalks, they can cause severe abdominal pain and vomiting.

Endometrial polyps: growths in the womb-lining which form on a stalk and can cause pain as they twist.

Endometritis: when the lining of the womb becomes somehow infected, for example by using an IUD.

4

Getting a diagnosis

Why is it important?

It is important to diagnose endometriosis because its treatment is different from that for other gynaecological or bowel problems. It is also thought that inflammation and scar-tissue build up each month, which can lead to further complications and also, in some cases, to infertility.

Having said that, other studies have shown that endometriosis doesn't always get worse. In fact, some research has shown that endometriosis can resolve itself spontaneously in 25 per cent of cases and can go from an active to a more passive form in 50 per cent of cases. The problem is that it is difficult to tell which women will get better and which will get worse.

So because endometriosis does seem to cure itself in some women, there is now an argument for not having treatment – especially if the endometriosis is mild. Whether or not to undergo treatment is a choice which an individual woman has to make after getting proper information about the condition. Some women decide they'll try anything to get rid of the pain, whereas others might want to start with the least drastic treatments and work their way from there.

Why are there delays in diagnosis?

There is an average delay of seven years from the onset of symptoms to getting a correct diagnosis. There are several reasons for this, one of the main ones being that women expect to get painful periods (one of the most common symptoms) so they aren't always aware that anything is wrong. Indeed, the 1995 NES survey revealed that over 50 per cent of respondents believed that their symptoms were normal. Also, women are often reluctant to seek help because they are embarrassed by the symptoms, especially if these include painful sex (30 per cent of women in the 1995 survey did not mention their experience of painful sex to their GPs).

What is more, doctors are not always very aware of endometriosis (57 per cent of women in the 1995 survey had been told at some stage that there was nothing wrong with them), and often confuse it with other conditions which have similar symptoms (see Chapter 3). It doesn't help that there isn't one specific symptom which relates solely to endometriosis. It can take a long time to rule out the other conditions first, and even when endometriosis is finally suspected there is often then a long waiting-list to see a specialist. There is also no specific test to diagnose endometriosis, other than visually by means of a laparoscopy.

> Paula says, 'I only found out I had endometriosis after one of my clients (I run a cleaning company) needed a cleaner because her endometriosis was making it difficult for her to do it herself. I went along, and by the end of the conversation I realized that I probably had endometriosis, too. Everything just sounded so familiar.'
>
> Jenny comments: 'It was my beautician who told me I had endometriosis. I was complaining to her that I felt tired all the time, had painful periods and sex when she suddenly cried, ''You've got endo!''. She then persuaded me to go back to my doctor and ask to see a gynaecologist. It was a good thing she did that, because endometriosis and fibroids were diagnosed and I eventually underwent a hysterectomy because of the pain.'

Dealing with doctors

Getting a referral

Unless you can afford to go privately, you have to be referred by your GP to a gynaecologist. When you visit your GP it is important that you are very clear about *all* your symptoms so that he or she can get a clear picture of what is wrong. It is therefore a good idea to make a list of your symptoms before visiting your GP or consultant. (It may help to read Chapter 3 to see if you recognize any of them.) If you feel very embarrassed you could even give the list to your GP to read. If doctors explain things in a very complicated way, don't be scared to ask them to repeat what they have said.

Many sufferers complain that their GP didn't take their symptoms seriously at first (over half the women in the 1995 survey thought that their GP didn't take their symptoms seriously, and 42 per cent thought that their GP was unhelpful). If this happens, don't be afraid to go back – often doctors operate a 'wait and see' procedure whereby they expect people to return if their problem is still troubling them. Other sufferers have complained that their doctor thought their condition was psychosomatic (all in the mind). Some women may be suffering from other problems, like depression, but that doesn't mean they aren't also suffering from endometriosis! Also, as we already know, endometriosis can be very exhausting leading to tiredness and depression.

Changing your GP

If you really feel your doctor isn't helping, you can ask to change doctors without giving a reason. To do this you just need to visit the surgery of your choice, taking along your medical card, and request to be taken on. The GP will either accept or refuse you. If you encounter any problems doing this you should ask either your local Community Health Council (CHC) or the Family Health Services Authority (FHSA) for help (their addresses are in the phone book).

Diane, 55, a practice nursing sister who eventually underwent a hysterectomy for endometriosis, says: 'My first GP wasn't at all sympathetic and when I eventually got hold of my medical notes I was horrified to see he'd written in a letter Munchausen's Syndrome with a question mark (a psychiatric condition where you purposely make yourself appear ill to attract attention). I couldn't believe he could say that when I'd already been diagnosed as suffering from endometriosis, and had had to have several operations. In those days you had to explain to your doctor why you wanted to change – so I went along with my husband to tell the GP I would be moving to another doctor whom I knew to be more sympathetic to endometriosis. During the discussion, I asked him why he'd written Munchausen's down. His only explanation was that he didn't really understand endometriosis. Although I did move, it makes me angry to think that it is still written down in my medical notes.'

How to get the best from your GP

1 Prepare for the consultation before you go. Think clearly about your symptoms and how they affect your life.
2 Make a list of your symptoms. You can actually take the list with you and read them out if you want.
3 Rehearse what you want to say, either with someone else or just in your own mind.
4 Take someone with you to the consultation for support. Everyone has a right to do this.
5 If you think you'll need longer than usual with your doctor, ask the receptionist if you can book a double appointment.
6 Take with you the names of any drugs or medicines you have been taking.
7 If the doctor suggests a physical examination, ask him or her what sort of information this might give. Also remember that you can ask for the examination to stop at any time if you're not happy.
8 If there's anything you don't understand, ask your doctor to explain – as many times as is necessary!

9 If you are prescribed any drugs, ask if there are any side-effects you should look out for.

10 If students are to be present at your consultation, the doctor should ask your permission first. You have the right to refuse.

11 If you want to see your medical notes, your doctor or practice manager can arrange this for you. You are allowed to see all your computerized records, but you can only see handwritten records made after 1 November 1991 (some doctors may still let you see these informally). If you have difficulty with this contact your local FHSA or CHC.

Making a complaint

Many practices have a complaints procedure which you can ask about at the reception. You can also issue an informal or formal complaint through your FHSA – though this must usually be done within 13 weeks of the incident. The CHC and FHSA can help you with this.

However, formal complaints can only be about your doctor's failure to fulfil the terms of his or her contract with the NHS. Complaints about their attitude are investigated informally with a non-medical person appointed by the FHSA to try and achieve some sort of reconciliation between doctor and patient. However, there is no compensation awarded through this procedure; you must contact a solicitor within three years of incident if you want to try for compensation.

Learning to be assertive

One of the problems we all have is not being assertive enough with our doctors. When you are feeling tired and run down or possibly depressed, it is much harder to stick up for yourself. If you are having problems with asserting yourself generally and asking for what you want, you could try taking an assertiveness course as an evening class or speaking to a counsellor of some sort (see Chapter 9).

Having said that, do still remember that your doctor is only human. He or she may have expertise or a special interest in conditions other than endometriosis. It will help enormously if you can give accurate information and are clear and polite about what you want to say.

Tests for endometriosis

The best way to diagnose endometriosis is to actually see it using a laparoscope. However, there are other tests which you might undergo before being referred for a laparoscopy, each of which is now described.

Physical examination

During a physical examination the doctor is looking for indications of possible endometriosis, such a pelvic mass (where organs feel as though they are matted together with scar-tissue) which may feel tender, or for adenomyosis or fibroids which may make the womb feel bulky. A physical examination may include:

- Feeling your abdomen on the outside to see if there is any tenderness, or if lumps can be felt through the abdominal wall muscles.
- Doing an internal examination to check that the vagina, womb and ovaries aren't tender or affected by lumps.
- Examining the rectum to check the ligaments (muscle bands of strong tissue) and to see if there are any lumps behind the womb.

But it is important to remember that, if the outcome of any of these examinations is that everything seems normal, it doesn't mean that you *don't* have endometriosis. You may also be asked to come back another time, because some problems don't show up until mid-cycle or just before or during your period.

Imaging techniques

The **ultrasound scan** is the main imaging technique used. It is completely harmless and is exactly the same device as is used to scan pregnant women. Some gel is put on to your stomach and a scanning head is then passed over your abdomen. It works by passing high-frequency sound waves through the body, which then bounce back to form an image of your pelvic organs on a computer screen. The problems with this method of diagnosis are that it can't distinguish between the different types of pelvic mass detected (i.e. whether it has found an endometrial deposit, a cyst or a tumour) and that it generally only shows up deposits of over two centimetres in size. It can be some help, though, in detecting whether the bowel or bladder is involved.

Other investigations

The Bowel

If your bowel is thought to be affected by endometriosis, you may have the following tests:

- **Digital rectal examination**: using a lubricated glove, a doctor examines the uterus ligaments using his finger and looks for lesions in the lower rectum. It is not usually painful, but can be a bit uncomfortable.

- **Barium enema**: during this procedure, the lower bowel is filled with fluid via a tube inserted into the lower colon through your rectum. This fluid is made of a substance which shows up on X-rays and reveals areas where there are any constrictions or unusual growths.
- **Flexible sygmoidoscopy**: a narrow fibre-optic tube is passed into your lower bowel via the anus. It allows the doctor to view the inner surface of the large bowel and to detect lesions. No anaesthetic is necessary, but it may feel a bit uncomfortable.

Grace had a digital rectal examination after being referred to a bowel specialist because she was suffering continual diarrhoea: 'I was asked to undress to the waist while the doctor left the room, and then to lie on my side on the bed with my knees up and my bottom exposed. He then came in and explained that he would be lubricating his finger and inserting it into my anus. Fortunately it didn't hurt, it just felt a bit uncomfortable. But it was all over very quickly and then he wiped the anus with a swab and gave me some disposable towels to clean away the lubrication.'

Karen, a 31-year-old hospital support worker, had to undergo a barium enema before endometriosis was diagnosed. She recalls: 'I was first given a muscle-relaxant injection into my vein which was supposed to slow down the gut and stop the bowel making spasms. It made me feel giddy and a bit sick. Then I had to lie on a table and a tube was inserted into my anus and up into my lower bowel. Air and then fluid was pumped into me via this thin tube. It did hurt quite a bit, but the medical staff treated me very well. I had to move around in different positions while they did the X-rays. Afterwards it took me a couple of days to recover from feeling bruised and windy!'

The urinary tract

These investigations include:

- **Kidney function tests**: to measure the amount of urea and salts in the blood, which can reveal whether your urinary system is involved.
- **Urinalysis**: a dip-stick test in a urine sample to exclude infection, kidney problems, diabetes and to detect urinary problems.
- **Urine microscopy**: a sample of urine is examined under a microscope for evidence of endometrial cells.
- **Urine culture**: urine is observed to see if any bacteria grow in it, which could indicate an infection.
- **IVU**: an iodine-based solution is injected into arm, enters the blood stream and is then X-rayed as it filters through the body to see if the kidney, ureter and bladder are functioning properly.

- **Cystoscopy**: a light anaesthetic is given, and a viewing device called a cystoscope is inserted into the bladder to look for any lesions, which are then biopsied (i.e. a small tissue-sample is taken for laboratory analysis). This is sometimes done during routine laparoscopy.
- **Hysteroscopy**: under local or general a anaesthetic, a camera is inserted into womb vaginally, to examine the lining.

Other blood tests

A sample of blood may be tested to look for evidence of infection or anaemia, or for evidence of inflammation or disease.

Future tests

Studies are still being carried out to develop a fool-proof blood test which would reveal whether a woman has endometriosis. It has already been discovered that women with endometriosis have a raised amount of a substance called CA125 in their blood, which is secreted by endometrial tissue. The problem is that this substance is also secreted by other women (such as those who are pregnant or have ovarian cancer). So it is impossible to tell without further investigation which condition is causing the rise.

Laparoscopy – the main test for endometriosis

What is a laparoscopy?

A laparoscopy is an operation to discover whether endometriosis is present in the pelvis. It involves having a small telescope-like device called a laparoscope – through which the surgeon looks – inserted through a small hole into your abdomen. In some cases, the laparoscopy is not just used to diagnose endometriosis but is also used to perform surgery to remove any endometriosis found at the same time (see Chapter 6 for more on surgery).

What happens during a laparoscopy?

The length of time you spend in hospital varies. Some hospitals do the treatment on an out-patient basis (i.e. your treatment takes less than a day and you can go home afterwards), whereas others may admit you for one to two nights.

You will not be allowed to eat or drink for 12 hours before the operation as you will be given a light general anaesthetic to put you to sleep throughout the operation. The reason for this rule is that eating or drinking could cause you to be sick during the operation, which could be dangerous or even fatal.

Once you are under anaesthetic, you are taken to the operating theatre, where carbon dioxide gas is pumped, via a small needle, into your abdomen. This helps to separate your pelvic organs from each other – particularly your womb and ovaries – and so makes it easier for the surgeon to look for signs of endometriosis.

A small incision (cut) is then made near your navel to insert the laparoscope, the surgeon's viewing device – it's rather like a telescope which magnifies everything. Another small incision may be made above your pubic bone, through which the surgeon's other instruments – such as a probe or biopsy forceps – can be passed, enabling him or her to look around properly. (Some surgeons use only the first hole for the whole operation passing both the laparoscope and surgical instruments through it.) A probe is a thin rod of pliable metal with a blunt swollen end, used for exploring cavities without causing abrasions. Biopsy forceps are metal pincers used to extract tiny pieces of tissue for a laboratory examination.

While this is going on, the surgeon's assistant inserts a probe into your vagina, and passes it through your cervix and up into the uterus to help the surgeon manipulate the womb in order to see more easily.

Any adhesions which are found are divided to allow the surgeon to see better – and also to relieve symptoms. This is usually done with scissors, or a heated cutting device called diathermy or a laser (see Chapter 6 for more detail).

The operating table is then gently tipped to allow the coils of the bowel to slip down, making it easier for the surgeon to inspect the following areas:

- ovaries;
- womb (uterus) wall;
- womb ligaments;
- Pouch of Douglas (the area behind the womb);
- colon and rectum (the colon is the main part of the large intestine which, as part of the digestive process, removes large amounts of water and certain minerals, and the rectum is the end of large intestine where faeces are stored);
- ovary ligaments;
- bladder surface;
- tubes running from the kidney to the bladder.

Any cysts found are drained, and biopsy samples are taken and sent for histology. Biopsy is the removal of small pieces of tissue, and histology is a microscopic examination of them, using staining techniques, to identify whether they are endometriosis cells. Some peritoneal fluid may also be drained and then analysed as an aid to diagnosis.

Finally the carbon dioxide gas is let out, the table returned to horizontal and the small incisions either stitched or stapled. The stitch may either dissolve or be removed by your GP.

After the operation

You may need to take painkillers afterwards because of the abdominal discomfort caused by the gas. There may also be some vaginal bleeding, so sanitary towels are usually advised as they reduce the risk of infection which sometimes occurs after an operation, and which tampons could contribute to. As well as this, some women experience nausea and tiredness because of the anaesthetic. Many women also complain of shooting shoulder-pains afterwards. These are caused by small amounts of carbon dioxide which are left behind and which collect under the diaphragm (the sheet of muscle between the abdomen and the chest) causing pain in your shoulders. This is called 'referred pain' – i.e. you experience it in a different part of the body from its cause.

Estimated recovery time

Doctors usually advise taking up to a week off work, but it is up to the individual concerned – some people may well need more time.

Maria recalls: 'I was given an information sheet which advised taking about three days off work. It also gave me the impression that I would get better very quickly.

Fortunately, I'd arranged for a friend to meet me in her car, because I would never have got home without her. I felt stiff, uncomfortable and could hardly walk. Once at home, I went straight to bed and slept for 24 hours. Luckily my friend stayed with me and was able to cook my meals – but really it took me more than a week to recover. So I think it is important to be well prepared!'

Danger signs

Very occasionally you can become ill after a laparoscopy, if your pelvic organs have been accidentally damaged. You should contact your doctor immediately if you experience any of the following:

- problems going to toilet
- smelly vaginal discharge or heavy bleeding
- feeling sick and vomiting
- fever or chills
- severe pain or increasing pain
- redness or swelling around the wounds.

What are the advantages of a laparoscopy?

- It's the only sure way to diagnose endometriosis, or to discover whether the cause is something else like PID (see Chapter 3);
- The diagnosis is accurate in 70 per cent of investigations;
- Only small incisions are needed, and so recovery is fairly quick.

What are the disadvantages?

- The surgeon has to be highly trained and experienced to be able to use the instruments effectively;
- It can trigger internal adhesions;
- Endometriosis can't always be detected by the human eye;
- It's not always possible to treat extensive problems with this method, so a laparotomy may be required (see Chapter 6).

Take note

If you have a negative laparoscopy and the pain persists it might be a good idea to press for a second laparoscopy.

'I had a laparoscopy'

Kim says, 'I've had five laparoscopies and have found that every surgeon has a slightly different procedure. For instance, sometimes I've stayed in overnight and at other times I've just been a day-patient.

Sometimes I've been asked to bath and shave my pubic hair before the op – but not always. Often I go in early in the morning, so I stop eating and drinking at midnight the previous night. There can be quite a lot of waiting around in the hospital, so I take my personal stereo and a relaxation tape to calm my nerves.

After having my chest listened to, and being asked questions like whether I've had operations before, I change into a surgical gown. Sometimes I'm given a pre-med which make me feel woozy; at other times I'm immediately given the anaesthetic. The surgeon sometimes says a few reassuring words before I go into the operating theatre.

After the operation, the surgeon tells me immediately what he has found. Because it's sometimes difficult to ask all the questions I want at this stage, I sometimes write them down – just the basics, like what did they find, what treatment they suggest, etc.

Generally, I recover quite easily and go back to work within a week. I don't get any abdominal pain at all, just a terrible shoulder-ache which is very common, and I take an over-the-counter painkiller to relieve it. When I find myself able to do household tasks like the ironing without getting tired, I know I'm back to normal.'

Classification of endometriosis

There are various systems used to classify different degrees of endometriosis, all of which calculate its severity according to a points system related to its internal distribution. The drawback with all of them is that they give points according to how far the disease is likely to affect your fertility, but don't take into account other considerations, like how much pain you are experiencing. Apparently there is a new American scale which does take these things into account, but it isn't yet in use over here.

The most common classification system used here was developed by the American Fertility Society in 1978, and revised in 1985. Using this system surgeons looks for lesions, nodules and cysts, giving points for each one found in specific areas and for their size. Adhesions are also counted on a rising scale depending on their nature, i.e. whether they are light or dense and whether they press into nearby healthy tissue. The extent of endometriosis is then usually described as **mild**, **moderate** or **severe**. Here are some examples of what this could mean:

Mild: Shallow deposits on the pelvic lining and on one ovary, with filmy adhesions on the other ovary.

Moderate: deep deposits on the pelvic lining and on one ovary; dense adhesions on the other ovary.

Severe: deep deposits on the ovaries, with dense adhesions on the ovary, Fallopian tube and pelvic lining.

The patches of endometriosis seen through the laparoscope vary greatly in appearance, and are commonly described in a number of ways:

- classic, gun-metal blue-grey spots;
- 'Raspberry' spots, with shaggy tissue at the edges;
- flat or raised white tissue, like scarring;
- clear 'berries' with small peaks;
- chocolate cysts filled with old blood.

These endometriosis deposits can be further classified according to the nature of their cells. The womb-lining normally has three different types of cells:

- surface cells;
- glands;
- stroma (the connective tissue which binds the glands together).

37

The more deeply embedded these cells are, the more difficult they are to remove. They can also be further graded according to their level of activity. Early, active cells usually have no colour, but when tested in the laboratory often have more biochemical activity than the older, darker-coloured areas of endometriosis, which can mean that they are more painful

Take note!

The main thing to remember is that, although your endometriosis may have been classified as mild, it may not *feel* mild, and needs to be taken just as seriously as a case of severe endometriosis which causes little pain.

5
Drug Treatments

How does drug treatment work?

There are many different types of drugs on the market for the treatment of endometriosis. But the main aim of all of them is to stop you having periods for six to nine months. The theory is that, once the patches of endometriosis are no longer stimulated by hormones released before or during your period, these patches will shrink and stop causing pain. Then, when your menstrual cycle returns to normal, endometriosis is less likely to occur.

The main hormone thought to stimulate endometriosis is the female sex-hormone oestrogen, and thus much of the treatment is aimed at reducing the amounts of oestrogen in your body. For this reason, too, many of the drugs prescribed for endometriosis aim to mimic the states of menopause or pregnancy. That's because, when a woman is pregnant or menopausal, she has smaller amounts of oestrogen in her body and endometrial deposits seem to regress.

Which drug should I take?

Obviously the best drug to take is the one which is the most effective for you and has the fewest side-effects. Side-effects vary from person to person, and the only way to find out what they are is to take the drug for a while. GPs usually recommend that you try a drug out for six months, but you are usually asked to return after three months to see how you are getting on. Allowing for the fact that your body is likely to take a little while to adjust when it is suddenly plunged into a state of false menopause or pregnancy, it's still a good idea to report any unwanted side-effects to your GP, if only to reassure yourself that they are normal.

However, if the side-effects are severe – such as raising your blood-pressure or causing tightness in your chest or changes in your voice – you should stop treatment immediately.

The effectiveness of the drug differs from person to person. Consultants usually suggest a drug which they think is suitable, based first on their opinions of endometriosis and second on their knowledge of any new drugs available. However, you don't have to agree automatically to take what your consultant suggests, and you can ask for a list of the side-effects before you decide. If, once you have tried a drug, you discover that it doesn't suit you, you can then go on to try others until you find the one you like best.

Most drugs used in the treatment of endometriosis are only licensed for six months use by a patient, and generally, if a drug hasn't worked in this time, it is unlikely to be of any help to you, and you might want to consider switching to another.

Warning: You shouldn't normally have drug treatment if you are pregnant, as it could cause foetal abnormalities. With most drug treatments, barrier methods of contraception should also be used to avoid pregnancy.

Remember that, with any drug treatment, you may experience no side-effects at all, or you may experience one or two side-effects – but it is very rare to have all of them!

What are the advantages of drug treatment?

- It can get rid of the pain! Drug treatment has been found successfully to treat pain in 85 per cent of cases.
- It can also get rid of any microscopic patches of endometriosis.
- It avoids the upheaval of going into hospital for surgery and the risk of post-operative adhesions (i.e. sometimes you get internal areas sticking together following surgery, because of the local inflammation this can cause).

What are the disadvantages of drug treatment?

- Drug treatment doesn't always get rid of large or deeply-embedded endometriosis.
- You may experience unpleasant side-effects.
- The long-term effects of drug treatment are not really known.
- It can be a hassle remembering to take tablets, nasal sprays or undergoing uncomfortable injections.

There follows a description of the various drugs prescribed for endometriosis, and some of the pros and cons of each.

1   The contraceptive pill

What is the contraceptive pill?

There are many different brands of the Pill on the market, some of the most common being Minilyn, Trinordiol, Logynon and Microgynon.

The combined contraceptive pill is often the first option suggested to an endometriosis sufferer, especially if you haven't started a family. It is the safest way to 'buy time', relieving the pain to a point where you might want to consider having children. Obviously, many young women don't know whether they want children at all, but it seems wise to keep options open if possible.

The combined contraceptive pill is basically made up of different combinations of oestrogen and progesterone, which has the effect of mimicking pregnancy, causing the lining of the womb, along with endometrial deposits, to shrink. When used to treat endometriosis, it's usually taken continuously and it's a good idea to take a low oestrogen or a progesterone-only Pill (because as we know, oestrogen encourages endometriosis).

Who takes it?

Any woman can take the Pill, but it is often prescribed to teenagers and young women with a mild form of the disease, and sometimes to women who have recurrent ovarian cysts. If you usually have no problems taking the Pill, it might be well worth considering.

Who can't take it?

- People with high blood-pressure;
- People who are at risk of developing blood clots;
- Smokers and women over 35 are more at risk if they take the Pill over a long period of time (as with normal contraceptive pills).

What dose should I take?

It's usually taken continuously for four to six months without the usual seven-day monthly break which you have when taking it for contraceptive purposes. If successful, it can be continued until a woman wishes to become pregnant or wants a 'natural' break.

What are the side-effects?

There are several, depending on the brand you take. But the commonly reported ones are generally:

- weight-gain
- nausea
- breast tenderness and enlargement
- depression
- headaches
- loss of sexual drive.

How successful is it?

It is thought not to be as effective as Progestogens, Androgens or GnRH analogues (see below). Many women find they have problems with breakthrough bleeding on the Pill, and say that it doesn't get rid of the pain. But it can relieve symptoms in some women and is certainly worth a try as the first option.

2 Androgenic drugs (male-type hormones)

What is danazol?

Danazol (marketed as Danol) was until recently the most common drug used for the treatment of endometriosis – the 1985 NES survey reported that 75 per cent of sufferers had taken it. A synthetic form of the male hormone testosterone, danazol works by making your body chemistry similar to a menopausal state, with low oestrogen and high androgen (male hormone) levels. It acts directly on the ovaries by interfering with the enzymes responsible for the production of the female hormones oestrogen and progesterone. As mentioned before, low amounts of oestrogen particularly discourage the growth of more endometriosis and help to shrink already established patches. It can also be used to treat women with breast disease, heavy periods and premenstrual syndrome.

One of the reasons doctors often prescribe danazol could be because it is relatively cheap compared to other treatments, such as Progestogens and GnRH analogues (more on these later).

Who usually takes danazol?

As well as to relieve pain, some women are given short courses of danazol before surgery to remove endometrial deposits thought to be causing infertility, or before undergoing a hysterectomy and removal of the ovaries. In both cases, the treatment aims to decrease the size and number of endometriosis patches to make surgery easier.

Grace says: 'I actually had drug treatment after I'd had surgery to remove fibroid and severe adhesions in my abdominal cavity. The consultant explained that it was to suppress my cycle for longer, and so to give my womb the best chance of recovering before my periods started again. I was a bit disappointed, though, when my periods returned, as they were still very painful.'

Who can't take danazol?

Women who:

- are pregnant or breast-feeding
- have a blood-clotting disorder called thromboembolic disease
- have male-hormone-dependent tumours
- have heart, liver or kidney problems
- have abnormal, undiagnosed, vaginal bleeding
- have porphyria (a rare metabolic disease).

What dose should I be on?

Women with mild endometriosis are usually given 400 mg a day; women with moderate to severe forms take up to 800 mg a day.

However, once your symptoms begin to clear up, the dose may be reduced. The drug is usually started on the first day of your period to make sure you're not pregnant. Although your periods usually stop when you take danazol, barrier contraception should also be used as a precaution because the drug can cause damage to the foetus.

What are the side-effects?

Many women stop danazol because of the side-effects, and three out of four women will notice at least one. The most common one reported by the NES is weight-gain (85%) – with the average gain being 4 kg (8.8 lb) by women taking the higher dose.

The other most common side-effects are:

- shrinking breasts (48%)
- oily skin (37%)
- flushing (42%)
- depression (32%)
- mood change (38%)
- sweating (32%).

Some of the side-effects, such as hot flushes and a dry vagina, are associated with being in a simulated state of menopause. Others are to do with making the body more male, such as increased hair and voice-changes. Only 7% of women reported voice-changes, but if it does occur you should stop the drug immediately as it can be permanent. Some sufferers also report joint-pain, although there's no official study on this.

Because danazol affects the blood-fats and liver function, it isn't a good idea to take it for a long time as there's no information on its long-term effects.

One of the symptoms widely reported, although not documented, is nausea.

> Joanne, a 27-year-old customer service supervisor who was diagnosed as having an endometriosis nodule between the bowel and the womb, says: 'I tried danazol for three weeks but it made me sick every day and there was just no way I could continue like that. So I switched to Zoladex and then went on to Synarel.'

How successful is it?

Many women's symptoms improve within four to eight weeks of starting the treatment, and over 85 per cent of women suffering from pelvic pain notice a significant improvement.

Women with mild endometriosis who want to get pregnant also have a better chance of conceiving.

Take note!

Weight-gain can be reduced by starting a diet-and-exercise programme before treatment. Many women have also found vitamin B6 and Evening Primrose oil (such as Efamol) can counteract some of the side-effects such as tiredness, depression, water retention and mood swings (more on this in Chapter 9).

3   Gestrinone

What is gestrinone?

Gestrinone (trade-name Dimetriose) is a synthetic hormone which has several different hormonal actions with characteristics of both male and female hormones.

How does gestrinone work?

It's not fully understood *how* gestrinone works, but it seems to act in two ways:

- It suppresses the release of the FSH and LH (see Chapter 1) from the pituitary gland. Without this stimulation to the ovaries, ovulation usually stops thus preventing the growth of endometriosis.
- It also seems directly to suppress endometriosis deposits.

What dose should I take?

As it lasts a long time in the body, gestrinone only needs to be taken twice a week – although this can sometimes be harder to remember than every day. Capsules usually come in 2.5 mg form, and are taken for six months.

Who can't take gestrinone?

Women who:

- are pregnant or breast-feeding;
- have severe heart, kidney or liver problems;
- have had metabolic or circulatory disorders during previous oestrogen or progestogen therapy. (The metabolism is the process by which the body makes use of its nutrients.)

What are the side-effects?

The main side-effects are:

- oily hair/skin
- muscle cramps
- fluid retention

- acne
- breast shrinkage
- itching.

Some trials have also suggested a weight-gain in 42 per cent of women taking gestrinone.

How successful is it?

Although it usually stops periods, spotting can occur. It seems to be as effective as danazol and MPA (see below). Some trials have suggested that there's a complete regression of endometriosis in 73% of women taking gestrinone.

4 Progestogens

What are progestogens?

Progesterone is a female hormone responsible for preparing the womb for pregnancy. In its synthetic form it can also cause the womb-lining to shrink and, along with it, any other endometrial deposits. 'Progestogen' is basically the name given to any substance which has the same effects as the natural hormone progesterone, and there are several different brands of progestogen on the market (listed below). Progestogens trick the body into thinking it's pregnant, resulting in a lowering of the levels of oestrogen in the body which helps relieve endometriosis. It's less commonly used than danazol, but is a useful alternative especially as the side-effects tend to be less severe.

Who can't take it?

As well as some of the general restrictions already mentioned with drug treatments (such as not being pregnant or breast-feeding), you should stop immediately if you experience any of the following:

- migraines
- pain or tightness of the chest
- jaundice
- itching
- high blood-pressure
- if you are due for an operation in the next six weeks.

There are also certain circumstances in which you shouldn't take a particular brand of progestogen – such as if you suffer from liver problems or thrombosis. You should always check with your GP before taking a drug to find out what these contra-indications are.

What dose should I be on?

It depends on the type of progestogen you are taking. The most common ones are **MPA** (trade-name **Provera**), **norethisterone** (several trade-names including **Primolut-N** and **Utovlan**), **dydrogesterone** (trade-name **Duphaston**) and the **progestin coil** (called **Mirena**. Let's now look at each of these in turn.

MPA

MPA (trade-name Provera) stands for medroxyprogesterone acetate; it is usually taken in the form of a 10 mg tablet three times a day for at least three months, but for not more than six months. In some cases, higher doses of up to 20 mg three times a day may be used. It's also available in injection form, known as Depo-Provera; this is usually used in cases of mild to moderate endometriosis.

Studies have shown that weight-gain tends to be lower than with danazol – with the average gain being 1.5 kg – but sufferers are likely to have more problems with fluid retention. Other side-effects include:

- heavier periods during the first few periods
- back-pain
- sore breasts
- bloating/fluid retention
- dizziness and headaches
- cramps
- irregular bleeding
- nausea
- lethargy.

When larger doses (of 100 mg or more per day) are used, it can also cause:

- milk-production from breasts
- gastric upsets
- hair-loss
- dry vagina.

> Fiona says: 'I put on several stone, and my breasts even began to produce milk! I got incredibly tired, and fell asleep as soon as I got home from work. But I did battle on, taking it for six months, because anything was better than dreadful period pains.'
>
> Ruth, a 29-year-old with endometriosis, says: 'I've been on Provera for a couple of years – first in tablet-form and now as an injection every 12 weeks. I've put on two stone in weight and find I get a very flaky scalp. I also suffered a bit from dizziness and nausea to start with, but that seems to have settled down. Apart from that, I'm quite happy with it.'

Take note: The side-effects are generally mild with Provera, but it must be taken with adequate medical supervision – especially as it can cause fluid-retention problems which may affect certain women, such as those with asthma, diabetes, epilepsy, renal dysfunction, depression and cardiac dysfunction.

Norethisterone

Norethisterone has several trade-names, such as Primolut-N or Utovlan. The dosage varies from 10 mg to 25 mg a day, for four to six months. The dosage is usually increased gradually until bleeding and spotting stops.

The side-effects include:

- nausea and bloating;
- exacerbation of epilepsy and migraine;
- possible change in liver-function (with higher doses);
- possible small rise in body temperature.

> Grace says: 'I felt awful on it. I suffered from dizziness, tiredness and found it hard to concentrate. I felt sort of spaced-out all the time, and not really like myself. I also got hot flushes and felt very depressed and anxious most of the time.'

Dydrogesterone

Dydrogesterone (trade-name Duphaston) is usually taken in daily doses of 10–30 mg for 6–12 months. In the doses generally used, it does not normally stop periods or ovulation. However, in some cases, gynaecologists may give higher doses of 30–60 mg daily, to stop menstruation. It can also be used in hormone replacement therapy (HRT), along with oestrogen, to counteract the side-effects of oestrogen.

The side-effects of dydrogesterone include:

- sore breasts
- irregular bleeding
- dizziness
- skin reactions

- bloating
- headaches
- nausea.

The progestin coil

Some women are now being treated with a coil called **Mirena,** which carries a progestin (a type of progestogen) used in oral contraceptives and HRT. It works by releasing a very low daily dose of the hormone directly into the womb. The coil itself also prevents the growth of the womb-lining and thickens the cervical mucus, which prevents the passage of sperm and suppresses ovulation in some women.

As the contraceptive pill is often the first line of treatment in the management of endometriosis, it may well be that coil could be equally effective. The makers say that, although it is not specifically licensed for the treatment of endometriosis, it is an option many gynaecologists are now considering.

Take note!

Generally progestogens seem to be as effective as danazol (sometimes slightly more so) but with fewer side-effects.

5   *GnRh analogues*

What are GnRH analogues?

GnRH analogues work by interfering with the action of a natural hormone called GnRH, which stands for gonadotrophin-releasing hormone. This hormone triggers the release from the pituitary gland of two other hormones – FSH (follicle stimulating hormone) and LH (luteinizing hormone) – which in turn set the menstrual cycle in action (see Chapter 1). GnRH analogues interfere with normal hormone production, causing periods to stop. Its effect is similar to that of removing the ovaries (only in this case it can be reversed!).

Who takes them?

GnRH analogues are available to most women, and are becoming more popular as the side-effects seem to be less severe than with other treatments.

Who can't take them?

Women who are:

- pregnant or breast-feeding;
- suffering from abnormal vaginal bleeding;
- allergic to the drug, or sensitive to other GnRH analogues.

See also the precautions of individual drugs listed below.

What dose should I take?

Unfortunately, GnRH analogues cannot be given by mouth, as they break down too quickly before having an effect. So they are usually taken in the form of nasal sprays, slow-release implants or as an intra-muscular injection. But they should not be taken if you are pregnant, and barrier methods of contraception should always be continued. The most common GnRH analogues are **buserelin** (trade-name **Superfact** or **Suprecur**), **goserelin** (trade-name **Zoladex**), **leuprorelin acetate** (trade-name **Prostap**) and **nafarelin** (trade-name **Synarel**), each of which we shall now look at in turn.

Buserelin

Buserelin (trade-name Superfact or Suprecur) is available as a nasal spray or injection. As well as treating endometriosis, it is also licensed for use in *in vitro* fertilization (IVF) programmes, because it stops a woman ovulating and thus losing the egg which must be collected for test-tube fertilization.

One spray of 150 mcg is usually taken in each nostril three times a day for six months. As well as the restrictions mentioned above, buserelin should be avoided if you have hormone-dependent cancers, and is also carefully monitored in women prone to depression as it can cause mood-changes.

The side-effects include:

- hot flushes
- mood swings
- nasal irritation
- loss of sex drive
- vaginal dryness
- sweats
- headaches
- break-through bleeding.

> Lesley says: 'I had a six-month course of buserelin nasal spray, and experienced side-effects of hot flushes, water retention and concentration difficulties, which worried me as I was taking a university course at the time. I found I had to read things over several times for them to sink in, and that I would often go upstairs to look for something and forget what I was looking for.'

(See also Helen's experience, described on p. 80.)

Goserelin

Goserelin (trade-name Zoladex) usually comes in an injection-form: 3.6 mg are injected once a month, for a period of six months, under the skin at the front of the abdomen, using a local anaesthetic. The goserelin is then gradually released into the body during the month.

Reported side-effects include:

- hot flushes
- headaches
- sweating
- mood changes
- loss of sex-drive
- depression
- dry vagina
- changes in breast-size.

Take note: Very occasionally women taking goserelin may enter the menopause, and never get their periods back afterwards. There is also a reduction in bone density during treatment, which can be partially reversed after treatment finishes. For this reason, women with a known metabolic bone disease are advised not to take it.

Karen, who took Zoladex for three months prior to laser surgery, says: 'Once a month I was given a local anaesthetic and then the Zoladex was injected into my belly, in the form of a little pellet. I did feel quite tender and bruised afterwards. The side-effects for me included hot flushes, a depressive feeling and night-sweats.'

Leuprorelin acetate

Leuprorelin acetate (trade-name Prostap SR) is administered once a month by the injection of a 3.75 mg dose into the arm, the abdominal wall or the thigh; injections continue for six months. It's sometimes prescribed to women 12 weeks before pelvic surgery.

The reported side-effects include:

- hot flushes
- insomnia
- loss of sex-drive
- nausea
- dry vagina
- loss of bone density
- weight-gain
- fluid retention
- mood changes
- headaches.

Nafarelin

Nafarelin (trade-name Synarel) is usually taken in the form of two 200 mcg sprays per day (400 mcg in total) for six months. Trials show that it works as well as danazol, but with a lower percentage of side-effects.

Side-effects may include:

- hot flushes
- mood swings
- dry vagina
- reduction in breast-size

- changes in sex-drive
- muscle pains

- headaches
- nasal irritation.

Linda says, 'I only took nafarelin for two months, but came straight off it because it gave me terrible headaches and made me feel very dizzy.'

Angela too found it unsuitable: 'It gave me mood swings and hot flushes, and I felt totally depressed on it, so I only took it for a month.'

Take note:

A lot of the side-effects of GnRH analogues are associated with menopausal symptoms, such as hot flushes, which occur in 74–98 per cent of women. One problem with these drugs is that the symptoms often get worse for a short time before they get better.

Many doctors are also worried about the long-term effects of thinning bones and the increased risk of heart attacks due to the lack of oestrogen when taking these drugs.

Ordinary menopausal women still have a certain amount of oestrogen which can protect them against these things. For this reason some doctors are prescribing a low dose of HRT to counteract the possible bone-thinning effects of these drugs. However, this can only be done at supervised centres where patients can be properly monitored. The NES should be able to provide more information on this (see Useful Addresses at the back of the book).

Why don't some treatments work?

Having drug treatment alone doesn't always work. This is because the drugs may have difficulty in attacking deeply embedded endometrial deposits, especially those which have glands and the ability to produce new endometrial cells and endometriomas (endometrial cysts on the ovary). Six months of treatment may also not be enough to be effective. For this reason, some women take lower doses for longer periods, or are happy to take the risk of being on treatment for longer. If in doubt, you should speak to your consultant on whether an option for you might be continuous medication with small breaks in between.

Less common drug treatments

What is Tamoxifen?

Tamoxifen is a drug which suppresses oestrogen and which is normally used to treat breast cancer. But it has also been known to shrink endometrial deposits and reduce pain in sufferers who haven't responded to other drugs.

The side-effects include:

- hot flushes
- acne

- constipation
- tiredness.

Painkillers for endometriosis

What is the best way to take painkillers?

It is a good idea to take painkillers with something which will line the stomach-wall – such as a meal, or a glass of milk and a biscuit. Never take them on an empty stomach!

Problems with painkillers

Often women with endometriosis don't find over-the-counter drugs very effective, especially as, over time, they seem to lose their effect.

However, it is not a good idea to take stronger painkillers, as prescribed by your doctor, for too long because they could become addictive. Many endometriosis sufferers find it is a good idea to juggle different strengths of painkillers around to suit their needs. For instance, they reserve the very strong ones only for very bad days. You should feel free to discuss with your doctor any painkillers you are taking which don't seem to be working. It might also be a good idea to investigate other, alternative methods of relieving pain (see Chapters 9 and 10).

What are the side-effects?

All painkillers can irritate the stomach-lining, causing nausea and vomiting, and in some cases lead to coughing-up or passing blood. Sometimes they can also cause constipation or diarrhoea.

Some of these side-effects can be offset by taking a simple anti-sickness tablet, such as a travel pill. Alternatively, you could try senna tablets which are a natural laxative, or lactulose, a manufactured syrup which speeds up the action of the gut giving extra lubrication to the faeces. Including fibre in your diet is also a good idea. As a general rule if, after trying a painkiller for two weeks, it has no effect, it is unlikely that it will help you and it would be worthwhile trying a different one.

Jacqueline says: 'At first I was given Ponstan [an NSAID–see below] for my endometriosis, which was only diagnosed by a pelvic examination. It did seem to reduce the heavy bleeding, but it irritated my stomach and made me feel very sick. I took it about twice a day for nearly two years until a new doctor who was reading up my notes said that I shouldn't have been on it for so long.'

We shall now look at the different painkillers available – both over-the-counter and prescribed drugs.

Over-the-counter painkillers

(NSAIDs: see under prescribed drugs below.)

Paracetamol: this acts as painkiller but isn't an anti-inflammatory. It is probably the easiest painkiller to take and has fewer side-effects than other analgesics (a more technical term for a painkiller). However, paracetamol may be less effective for more than mild pain.

Aspirin: reduces inflammation and fever, but can cause stomach irritation so should be taken with food or milk, or as a soluble tablet. It is good for mild to moderate pain.

Ibuprofen: another popular anti-inflammatory or NSAID. It's a mild painkiller but it can also irritate the stomach.

Feminax: this is one of the various anti-spasmodic drugs on the market, specifically for period pain; but it can cause nausea and drowsiness.

What is DLPA?

DLPA is a nutritional painkiller which is a mixture of two forms of phenylalanine – an amino acid found in food proteins.

How does it work?

If taken regularly, DLPA is thought to protect and strengthen our body's own natural painkillers (endorphins). Because phenylalanine is one of the eight essential amino acids which occur naturally in our bodies, DLPA isn't classed as a drug but rather as a nutritional supplement. It has been found to help with acute and chronic pain, and also with lower back-pain, premenstrual cramps and joint pains, among other things.

How do you take DLPA?

DLPA tablets are usually taken for several weeks rather than just at the time when you are experiencing pain. The dose is usually 375 mg capsules (i.e. two capsules) three times a day at meal-times. Once you start to feel the painkilling effect, you can either reduce the dose or stop taking them until the next time you need them.

What are the advantages of DLPA?

- It can have an effect equal to taking morphine, but isn't addictive;
- It can be used in conjunction with drugs and other therapies such as acupuncture;
- It helps with the depression which often accompanies chronic pain;

- Pain relief can continue for up to a month after stopping the treatment.

What are the disadvantages of DLPA?

- It doesn't work for everyone – 30 per cent of users get little or no relief;
- It can cause severe indigestion;
- It shouldn't be taken if you are pregnant, if you suffer from high blood-pressure or are on monoamineoxidase inhibitor drugs for depression.

Lesley says: 'I've found I have absolutely no side-effects with DLPA, and I'm very happy with it. I usually take it over three weeks and find that it provides pain relief for the following three months.'

Prescribed painkillers

If over-the-counter painkillers don't work, your doctor might prescribe any of the following stronger painkillers.

Mild to moderate strength: co-analgesics, such as codydramol or solpadol, which are a mixture of codeine and paracetamol. Distalgesics such as coproxamol, which contain a mixture of dextropropoxyphene and paracetamol, are also of a similar strength.

Moderate to strong: dihydrocodeine, also known as DF118, and nefopan are both moderate to strong painkillers, but can cause constipation and dependency.

The strongest: opiates or opioids, such as morphine and pethidine. (Drugs such as Fentanyyl are synthetic version of these.) These are only prescribed for severe pain, and are not suitable for long-term use as you can become dependent quickly, even in low doses.

Tranquillizers, sleeping pills and anti-depressants: these may also be prescribed for chronic pain. They include diazepam – a form of valium – and carbemazepine, an anti-anxiety drug which can control muscle spasms and which may be used for nerve pain.

NSAIDS

NSAID stands for 'non-steroidal anti-inflammatory drug'; trade-names include Ponstan, Apsifen, Brufen, Naprosyn, Synflex, Laraflex and Votorol. NSAIDs are a mild type of painkiller which work by inhibiting the production of prostaglandins in the body. They can be bought over-the-counter, though the stronger versions are only available on prescription.

Prostaglandins are chemicals made by body-tissues; they send 'messages' to the womb causing it to shrink, and also cause the womb-walls to contract during periods or childbirth. They're also part of the body's natural healing mechanism, as they go to the sites of injury and activate its pain-receptors, causing inflammation. It's thought endometriosis sufferers have extra prostaglandins because these can be produced by endometriotic tissues.

The idea behind NSAIDs is that, if you introduce drugs which block prostaglandins, you will suffer less pain. However, they work best if they are taken early on in the pain-cycle. For instance, if you know you usually experience pain on Day 21 of your menstrual cycle, it's a good idea to start taking them the previous day.

6
Surgery

What is surgery?

Surgery is the branch of medicine which treats disease or injury by an operation involving cutting or manipulating the infected parts. There have been a lot of recent surgical developments for the treatment of endometriosis – but unfortunately there are no studies on whether surgery is more effective than drug treatment. The decision whether or not to have surgery needs careful consideration, and should be based on your individual situation – such as how bad your endometriosis is and whether you've had children already. Surgery is often used in conjunction with drug treatment, which is often given before an operation to reduce the number of endometrial deposits requiring surgery.

Surgery for endometriosis is divided into the following two categories:

Conservative surgery: this is when patches of endometriotic tissue, cysts and adhesions are removed leaving your organs intact, so that it is still possible for you to become pregnant. The operations are laparoscopy (see Chapter 4), laparotomy, laser laparoscopy, microsurgery – all described later in this chapter.

Definitive or radical surgery: when your womb, Fallopian tubes and ovaries are taken out – and it is no longer possible to become pregnant. These operations are described in Chapter 7.

Why have surgery?

Surgery is usually advised in the following situations, when:

- drug treatment hasn't worked;
- your symptoms have returned after drug treatment;
- reconstruction of an organ is needed as treatment for infertility;
- your endometriosis is severe, and includes adhesions and is affecting other important organs such as the bowel or intestines;
- your family is complete;
- you specifically request surgery.

What are the advantages of surgery?

- It's the only way to remove large, deeply embedded patches of endometriosis, cysts and adhesions;

- there are no side-effects, as with drugs;
- the treatment can result in immediate pain relief;
- new methods, such as laser surgery, are now so improved that there is minimal risk of the damage which was sometimes caused during conventional surgery (such as causing adhesions).

What are adhesions?

Adhesions are a type of scar-tissue which forms inside the body when the lining of the abdominal cavity is injured or inflamed, either by infection, surgery or even endometriosis itself. The strands of these adhesions can sometimes stick pelvic organs together.

What are the disadvantages of surgery?

- It requires time off work for the surgery and recovery;
- you have to undergo an anaesthetic;
- the surgeon can only remove what he or she can see (so microscopic deposits of endometriosis can't be removed);
- it's sometimes difficult to recognize endometriosis;
- the endometriosis may be close to sensitive organs, such as the bowel, and can't be removed for fear of damaging the organ;
- surgery might cause worse damage – it can cause more adhesions which can reduce fertility;
- endometriosis may still recur.

There now follows a description of the operations involved in conservative surgery.

1   Laparotomy

What is a laparotomy?

A laparotomy is a major operation to open the abdomen, remove endometrial sites and correct any other problems with the reproductive organs. It's often abbreviated to CSEL, which stands for conservative surgery for endometriosis at laparotomy. It's not as popular as it used to be because of the development of laparoscopy (see Chapter 4), but is still considered suitable if:

- you have experienced complications during a laparoscopy;
- you suffer from severe endometriosis and adhesions;
- you need more extensive work done on other organs;
- you are overweight, which can make a laparoscopy difficult.

What happens during a laparotomy?

You undergo a general anaesthetic, after which a 10–15 cm cut is made below the bikini-line (the scar later fades). Any ovarian cysts or patches of endometriosis are removed, and adhesions are separated and removed if possible. This is done by using either heat treatment, incisions or laser. During the operation, a procedure called presacral neurectomy may also be carried out if you suffer from severely debilitating pain. This involves cutting a bundle of non-essential nerves, so that some of the pain-messengers from the pelvis no longer reach the brain. However, this can only be done with your consent, and its results so far have not been very successful, so it is advisable only as a last resort.

What are the advantages of a laparotomy?

- Open surgery gives the surgeon a better view of your pelvic organs;
- there is less risk of damage to other organs;
- laser surgery can also be used during the operation;
- it alleviates pelvic pain in 80 per cent of cases, and in women suffering from infertility, the pregnancy rate after a laparotomy is 52 per cent.

What are the disadvantages of a laparotomy?

- Because of the larger cut, there is more risk of adhesions forming afterwards;
- there is a longer recovery time and a more extensive scar than with a laparoscopy;
- if extensive surgery is needed, there's more risk of infection and damage to the pelvic organs;
- endometriosis recurs within five years in 35 per cent of women who have undergone a laparotomy.

'I had a laparotomy?

Grace went in for a laparoscopy but then proceeded to a laparotomy because it was difficult to remove the dense adhesions.

She says: 'I think I was in the operating theatre for quite a long time as I went in at 2 p.m. and didn't wake up until 8 p.m. They told me then that I'd had extensive endometriosis on my womb and ovaries, and that this had been lasered off and the adhesions removed. But unfortunately they had to leave an adhesion which was sticking my womb to the bowel because they were worried about damaging the bowel.

When I woke up I had a scar about seven inches long. I also had a small blood transfusion going into one arm because I'd lost so much blood, and an antibiotic drip in the other arm. I also had a deep stomach drain coming out of the scar which drained debris into a bottle beneath my bed.

I had a catheter in place too, which gave me the feeling that I was going to the loo all the time, but as soon I got used to it they took it out. I was in hospital for six days, during which time I had painkilling injections of pethidine every three hours.

I was told it would take me about six weeks to recover and that I shouldn't lift anything heavy until then, and so I arranged for friends to do my shopping for me. Within three weeks I was mobile again and able to walk around. It did take three weeks, though, for the pain to go away.

All in all I'd say it took me about ten weeks to recover. Fortunately I'd arranged everything well, making sure people could come in and see me and help me with the housework. I also cleaned the house from top to bottom before going in to make it easier for me when I came out.

I did feel a bit depressed afterwards, as though I'd been violated because someone had touched my insides, and I had a few flashbacks of the operation. No one tells you about that!'

2   Laser laparoscopy?

What is a laser laparoscopy

The word laser is an abbreviation for light amplification by stimulated emission of radiation. Various substances give out a very thin beam of light when they are stimulated by an electrical charge. This beam of light can then be controlled using mirrors, and directed down a laparoscope very precisely on to one area to burn away or vaporize (a type of melting) endometrial tissue. These lasers are so accurate that it is possible for them to cut grooves into a human hair. Because they are so precise, they cause no damage to surrounding tissues during treatment.

There are four main types of laser:

- the carbon dioxide laser: used for treating mild to moderate endometriosis because it is easy to control;
- the argon laser: for vaporizing (melting) large cysts and sealing blood vessels;
- the KTP (potassium titanyl phosphate) laser: penetrates deeply and so is good for treating large, deeply embedded cysts which are difficult to get at;
- the nd-YAG (neodymium – yttrium aluminium garnet) laser: used to destroy large deposits because it penetrates deeply into tissues.

What happens during a laser laparoscopy?

As well as the two usual cuts which are made during a laparoscopy (through which the laparoscope and the handling instruments are passed, as described in Chapter 4), two more tiny incisions are made on either side of the abdomen, below the bikini-line. One is for the laser and the other for the venting device which allows waste-gases and tissue out of the abdomen and through which fluid is passed to wash out the cavity. The laser is then used to divide adhesions, vaporize deposits of endometriosis, drain cysts and improve fertility by reconstructive surgery.

As with a laparoscopy, these incisions are closed afterwards with a single stitch or staple. The procedure may also involve the division of uterine nerves with a laser, often referred to as LUNA (laser uterine nerve ablation) which stops some of the pelvic pain-messages getting to the brain.

Jackie says, 'When I had my second laser laparoscopy because of severe endometriosis, they also did LUNA treatment to help with the pain relief – and the symptoms did improve for a while. Afterwards I'd get a deep, strong aching pain around this area when walking or exercising. I also found I experienced some pain on orgasm afterwards. However, my symptoms did generally improve for a while.'

What are the advantages of a laser laparoscopy?

- Laser burns heal very quickly with minimal scar-tissue and bleeding;
- there is less disruption to your life because a laser laparoscopy can usually be done during a 24–48-hour hospital stay;
- it has a 70 per cent success rate in relieving abdominal pain;
- it can increase your chances of pregnancy, sometimes as much as 75%.

What are the disadvantages of a laser laparoscopy?

- New lesions can form at new sites after treatment;
- there's a small risk of damage to the bowel, bladder or blood vessels when the laparoscope is inserted or if a laser is inaccurately used, which can lead to the need for a laparotomy to correct them;
- surgery may be no more effective than drug treatment.

How can I get this treatment?

Your consultant will usually advise if he or she thinks that laser treatment is suitable for you. However, not all hospitals have laser equipment, in which case you could ask to be referred to one that does. It is then up to your own area health authority whether they are willing to pay the cost of sending you there. The NES should be able to help you with a list of recommended hospitals (see Useful Addresses at the back of book).

'I had a laser laparascopy'

Vanessa says: 'After a laparoscopy and two scans revealed that one of my ovaries was inflamed, I was admitted for laser surgery at Queen Charlotte's Hospital in Chelsea, for two days. After being visited by just about everyone – the surgeon, the anaesthetist and so on – I was given an anaesthetic and taken down to the operating theatre. I believe I was in the operating theatre for about five hours.

I woke up to find two incisions around my navel area and a third on the right-hand side of my stomach. I must admit, the pain was terrible. I was told it would take two weeks to recover, but really it took me over six. I felt such a wimp about it! My mother had to look after me for the following two weeks because I could hardly move from my bed because of the pain. She even had to wash my hair for me!

I also had to wear a sanitary towel because of the bleeding from the laser sites. I was relieved, though, that they had found some endometriosis because my previous consultant had been very sceptical. They found it in front of and behind my womb, and said they had just got to it in time before it spread to my ovaries! I was pain-free for five months, but unfortunately it then returned and so I'm going to have the operation repeated.'

3   Microsurgery

Microsurgery is a new technique, still being researched, and involving special teflon-coated metal tools which don't cause abrasions and adhesions because of their non-stick surface. Incisions are made with a hot wire which cuts as well as seals, and the 'debris' is then removed by suction. The procedure is highly methodical involving very neat stitching, which works well for separating adhesions and not replacing them with new ones. Sometimes artificial patches are used to prevent organs sticking together again. The other advantage of this method is that there is slightly less of a risk of infection occurring afterwards.

Lynn had three hours of microsurgery to separate adhesions and cauterize the endometriosis, after getting advice from the National Endometriosis Society on a surgeon who specialized in this procedure. She says, 'I found it didn't hurt as much after microsurgery as with ordinary surgery. The sites also definitely healed quicker and I wasn't in so much pain.'

Operations: general hints and tips

What to ask before any operation

It is important to ask your consultant exactly what sort of operation you are undergoing, and to have anything explained which you don't understand. You might also want to find out the following:

- How long will you stay in hospital, and how long will it take to recover?
- What action will be taken if complications occur, i.e. will a laparotomy then be carried out? When signing the operation consent form, you can ask that a hysterectomy and/or the removal of the ovaries should not be performed.
- What symptoms can you expect afterwards?
- Is the surgeon fully trained in laparoscopic techniques, and does he or she hold a certificate in this? (You will have to be tactful, perhaps asking how successful the surgeon finds this treatment, or something along those lines!).

Take note!

It is important to be sure, before surgery, that you are not pregnant. If in doubt, you should undergo a pregnancy test.

Tips on preparing for an operation

Elizabeth's preparations before having surgery to remove an endometrial lump in the hernia area may be helpful.

She says: 'I couldn't find any one book on what to do before going in for an operation, so I gathered information from all over. I increased my vitamin intake – Evening Primrose oil, vitamin E and a multi-vitamin tablet. I took as many gentle walks and swims as I could and carried on working, which I really enjoy.

I also had more regular acupuncture to help me cope with the pain and to boost my immune system and I used affirmations from Louise Hay's book (listed at the end of the book) writing my favourite one on a photo to take with me. I also wrote down as many questions as possible to ask the hospital staff, took the painkillers I'd been given and ate lots of good food, relaxed and started taking herbal remedies – Rescue Remedy and arnica tablets – a week before surgery.

I packed the following in my bag:

- a new dressing gown and night-shirt
- a personal stereo with a tape of relaxing music

- some lavender essence
- arnica tablets and Rescue Remedy
- a book of short stories
- a few other bits the hospital suggested, such as a towel and moisturiser.

Then, once I was in hospital, I created my own environment by my bed: I put a photo on the table and a few drops of lavender essence on the pillow, and had music playing quietly. One of the nurses smelt the lavender and came to chat about an aromatherapy course she'd done. Someone else promised me she'd be there when I woke up, and the nurse who shaved me did it with so much humour and dignity that it made everything bearable. They even let me take my music softly playing all the way to the operating theatre, and when I woke up someone had started it playing and put it beside me.

I can't pretend it was all smooth sailing. I didn't come out of the anaesthetic very well. However, the nurses were wonderful, one held the bowl for me while I was sick as another rubbed my back. The nurse who had done the aromatherapy also came to massage my feet and hands gently later on. I was amazed to receive such loving care. I stayed overnight and the next day went home.

I was off work for five weeks in the end – longer than I had anticipated. This was partly due to the constipation caused by the painkillers. This is no joke and I would recommend plenty of fruit, in particular stewed apples or cooked tomatoes, to ease this.

One of the pages in a scrapbook I made also contained a list of things to look forward to, such as a friend's wedding, my brother's baby and a class in pottery. Certainly focusing on this helped me to plan ahead, as well as accept my daily progress. My colleagues sent me a large bowl of plants – which made me take a daily walk to and from the kitchen to water them!

I also had a few meals ready prepared in the freezer, and my family were very helpful getting shopping and giving lots of love and changing sheets. The key is to be organized!'

What to ask after the operation

When you have recovered from your operation, it is important to ask the surgeon exactly what has been done. This is often done at a follow-up appointment, if not at the time. But even then, women are often given insufficient information about their problem. You might want to avoid this by at least asking the following questions:

- What degree of endometriosis was found?

- Were there any adhesions?
- Were your bowel or reproductive organs affected in any way?
- Is any further treatment needed?
- What are the advantages and disadvantages of this treatment?

It might be well worthwhile making a list so that you don't forget!

7

Hysterectomy

General information

What is a hysterectomy?

Hysterectomy means the surgical removal of the womb. It is either done through an incision in the abdominal wall or vaginally. About 15 per cent of women in Britain have had a hysterectomy, usually because of heavy periods (one of the symptoms of endometriosis).

Why have a hysterectomy?

A hysterectomy is usually only advised for older women who have already completed their family – although some young women with severe endometriosis do opt for it (normally only when all other treatments have failed). It is usually advised in the following circumstances:

- if your womb is getting bigger causing you circulatory problems or difficulties going to toilet;
- if you have severe pelvic pain;
- if you haven't responded to other treatments;
- if the quality of your life is severely affected.

What are the advantages of having a hysterectomy?

- It can greatly relieve endometriosis pain;
- you no longer have to put up with PMS and heavy periods;
- it may increase your sex-drive because you are no longer plagued by pain – and some women even say their orgasms improve!
- you no longer need to use contraceptives;
- it can mean a new life.

What are the disadvantages?

- It isn't reversible;
- it can affect your sex-life adversely – some women complain of less sensation during orgasm;
- if your ovaries are removed suddenly, you immediately become menopausal, which can lead to depression, lowered sex-drive and problems associated with the menopause, such as vaginal dryness (see later);

- even when the ovaries remain, some women may experience the menopause slightly earlier following a hysterectomy;
- you may suffer emotionally because of loss of your child-bearing ability.

For instance Irene, who had a hysterectomy at 38, recalls: 'Afterwards I found myself looking wistfully at little children, and went through a sort of mourning for the loss of my ability to conceive.'

What should you bear in mind when deciding?

It is a good idea to have counselling before and after a hysterectomy. Studies show that women who make the decision themselves tend to suffer fewer emotional problems afterwards. If you are nearing the menopause anyway, you might also decide you would prefer to wait for it to occur naturally. You should contact your GP for information on counselling.

What happens during a hysterectomy?

Here is a description of the main types of hysterectomy:

A total abdominal hysterectomy (TAH)

A TAH is when your whole womb and cervix are removed. It usually involves having just a bikini-line incision, but where there are other complications – like ovarian cysts or a previous vertical scar such as a Caesarean – a vertical scar may be needed instead. You are also given a catheter, a flexible tube which is inserted into the bladder during the operation to drain away urine; this may stay in place for a few days afterwards so you don't have to worry about going to the loo (some women say this can feel quite uncomfortable).

The surgeon then carefully cuts the womb away from its ligaments and blood vessels, and seals them up by clamping them off. If you are keeping your ovaries, the Fallopian tubes will also be separated from the womb and clamped off. The cervix is then cut away from the vagina, which frees the womb, allowing it to be lifted out and sent for examination. The hole where the cervix was is then stitched up. If the ovaries are to be left, they may be stitched to the pelvic wall to avoid the possibility of them getting in the way during intercourse. Sometimes a drain is left in for a few days to suck out any remaining debris or blood. Usually your stay in hospital lasts a week – or longer, if any complications occur.

'I had a hysterectomy'

Christine, who is 36 with two children, says: 'I went in the day before the hysterectomy and had all the usual checks done. Then from midnight I wasn't allowed anything to eat or drink. In the morning I was given a pre-med and taken to the operating theatre. I think it took about an hour-and-a-half, and when I woke up I cried with relief. I felt peaceful and restful, and no longer all twisted up inside. I couldn't stop thanking the medical staff!

I had a special drip going into my arm, with a button I could press to give myself painkillers, and I had an oxygen mask nearby because I was a bit faint. After that, I slept most of the day. Fortunately I was able to pass urine, though they give you a catheter if you had difficulty. I was also given a mild laxative to help me go to the loo. They taught me to cough with a rolled-up towel in front of my abdomen so that I wouldn't strain the scar.

The wound site had a drain on it and the stitches were very well done (coming out in one go after just three days). I found my appetite gradually returned, but for the first six weeks I couldn't do much. Friends from my local church helped me out at home. But it took me a good six months before I felt calmed down and stable.

I'm really glad I had the hysterectomy, as I've put on over a stone in weight since (I was too thin before), and now I only get twinges of pain whereas before I was in pain all the time. I used to have to fight just to make my children's sandwiches. I remember my small daughter seeing me in bed all the time, saying, ''Poor mummy, in bed all the time''. Now she's got the chance to have a real mummy who can even do the hoovering!'

A sub total or partial hysterectomy

This is where the womb is removed while the cervix is left in place. The advantage of this is that it is an easier operation to perform, and there is less risk of complications afterwards. It may also be carried out if the cervix is too difficult to remove, due to adhesions. However, women who have had this operation still need cervical smears, as they are still at risk of cervical cancer.

Wertheim's hysterectomy

Usually this is only performed in cases of cancer, but it is occasionally used to treat advanced endometriosis. It involves a more widespread removal – not just of the womb and cervix, but also of the uterine broad ligament, ovaries, Fallopian tubes, plus any lymph glands and fatty tissues at risk.

Jennifer, 48, underwent a Wertheim's hysterectomy when she was 40, after the discovery of endometriosis which was partially blocking her bowel, and because of multiple small cysts on the ovary. She says: 'When I had the hysterectomy I couldn't understand why the other women in the ward were recovering more quickly than I was. Then the consultant explained that the endometriosis had been so bad that he'd had to take out everything he possibly could, including the ligaments, and that the whole operation had involved 200 internal stitches. So it was no wonder I felt so ill!'

Vaginal hysterectomy

A vaginal hysterectomy means that the whole operation is performed through the vagina, so there is no abdominal scar. It is also supposed to mean a shorter stay in hospital (of three to five days, as opposed to four to seven days for a TAH) and a quicker recovery time (five weeks, as opposed to six to eight weeks for a TAH). The vagina may also be tightened during the operation, and the bladder treated for stress-incontinence. However, this operation isn't suitable for women who have dense adhesions.

The laparoscopically assisted hysterectomy

This is a vaginal hysterectomy carried out using a laparoscope, the viewing device described in Chapter 4. With this technique, three small cuts are made in the abdomen, through which the viewing device and the surgeon's instruments are passed. The stomach is also pumped with gas to help the surgeon see the organs more clearly. During the operation the surgeon may also divide any adhesions, as well as cutting away the uterus and ovaries (if necessary). The gas is then expelled, and the womb and ovaries removed through the vagina.

Should I have my ovaries removed?

Removal of the ovaries is known as an 'oophorectomy' if one ovary is removed, or a 'bilateral oophorectomy' if both are removed. The operation is an even more serious undertaking than those described previously, because it causes the immediate onset of the menopause. Nevertheless, a lot of endometriosis sufferers choose to have their ovaries removed because this is more likely to rid them of their pain by stopping the monthly cycle. The reason for this is that the ovaries produce oestrogen – one of the main female hormones which stimulates the patches of endometriosis.

So your womb might be removed and you may no longer have periods, but if your ovaries remain, any remaining patches of endometriosis can still be stimulated every month, causing pain and sometimes also creating the same period-like symptoms, such as PMS, stomach cramps and so on. Women who have had a hysterectomy but whose ovaries have remained have a 13 per cent chance of endometriosis recurring within three years.

Many women say that losing their ovaries is even more traumatic than losing the womb.

Sally recalls: 'I wasn't so upset about losing my womb because I had two children and I'd already been sterilized, but I was upset about losing my ovaries. I felt as though I had lost my femininity and went through a phase of wearing lots of very heavy make-up to try to compensate for it. Fortunately, though, this feeling began to fade over time.'

After the operation

Hysterectomy is a relatively safe operation with a death-rate of only six women in every 10,000. But studies show that complications occur in between 25 and 50 per cent of cases – these are mostly minor (such as urinary tract infections, urinary retention, pelvic abscesses, pain on intercourse). The more serious complications include haemorrhages, damage to other organs and blood clots (but these are very rare!).

Recovery time

Doctors advise you not to lift things for at least six weeks after the operation, and say that it will take up to eight weeks to recover.

Jennifer recalls: 'I was in hospital for eight days, but I found that I could walk around almost immediately after the operation, though only very slowly. I could also do things like make myself cups of tea, but I would get tired very quickly. For the first few weeks I'd get up for a couple of hours and then go to bed again in the afternoon. My daughters came in to help with the housework, and a neighbour did the ironing. But I made the mistake of trying to go shopping in the supermarket four weeks after the op. and ended up collapsing. I went back to work after three months, but really I think to recover fully I should have had four months off.'

Every woman is different, so don't worry if you need longer for your recovery time. You also need to allow time for the emotional adjustment: many women report it taking up to a year to get used to living without a womb.

When can I have sex again?

Many women worry about when they will be able to resume their sex-life. Again this varies, although doctors say as soon as the discharge and swelling have settled down, or after your first six-week clinic check. The simple rules are:

- don't hurry – take your time;
- stop if anything hurts;

- experiment with different positions to find out which is comfortable;
- use gels, such as KY jelly, and pessaries if you have lubrication problems;
- pelvic exercises and live fresh yoghurt applied to the vagina is also supposed to help (see Chapter 9 on pelvic exercises).

What is the menopause?

The menopause, often referred to as 'the change of life', is the time when your last period occurs. This is seldom clear-cut: periods can come and go for a few years after the first irregularity in your cycle. The menopause is the result of the ovaries running out of eggs; for most women, this happens between the ages of 45 and 55. If you've had a hysterectomy and your ovaries have been left in place, you may be one of the 25% of women who experience menopausal symptoms within two years of having the operation. But when both ovaries are removed during surgery, the menopause usually occurs very rapidly.

What are the symptoms?

Most of the symptoms are related to the withdrawal of oestrogen and the effect of increasing levels of the FSH (see Chapter 1) which result. The most common symptom is **hot flushes**, experienced by nearly 80 per cent of women. Other often immediate effects include night sweats and needing to go to the loo a lot.

Self-help for hot flushes

- Wear lots of layers of light clothing which can be easily removed and replaced.
- Avoid synthetic materials because these prevents the air from circulating freely.
- Cut down on caffeine drinks, alcohol, spicy food and smoking – all of which are thought to trigger flushes.
- Try frequent lukewarm showers rather than a bath.
- Exercise regularly
- Take vitamin E (200–400 international units each day), which is supposed to help excessive flushing and sweats.
- Try any of the capsules now on the market containing trace elements and vitamins especially for the menopause.
- For night sweats, place a cotton towel over your lower bed-sheet to absorb extra perspiration.

More long-term effects include dryness of the vagina and skin generally, a loss of sex-drive, and intercourse problems due to the thinning of vaginal walls, making them sore and susceptible to tearing.

Hormone replacement therapy (HRT)

What is HRT treatment?

Hormone replacement therapy (HRT) involves taking, in synthetic form, some of the hormones which your ovaries have stopped making (normally oestrogen and progesterone).

Why take HRT?

- It can relieve some of the symptoms of the menopause.
- It helps prevent osteoporosis – a thinning of the bones caused by calcium leaching from them, caused by a lack of oestrogen.
- Research has shown that it could offer some protection against heart attacks and strokes.

What are the risks of HRT?

Women have been having HRT for over 20 years, and evidence shows that it is safe for most women. However, it is important to tell your doctor that you have endometriosis (this will affect the drugs prescribed) or if any of the following apply to you:

- You or any of your close family have had breast cancer
- you have had cancer of the womb or ovaries
- you've had large fibroids
- you have active endometriosis
- you have a history of thrombosis or blood clots
- if you are a heavy smoker.

Or if you suffer from any of the following:

- severe migraine
- high blood-pressure
- diabetes
- liver disease
- gallstones
- a form of skin cancer called malignant melanoma

- otosclerosis (an ear condition)
- multiple sclerosis
- porphyria (a hereditary disease).

What are the disadvantages of HRT?

Many women report unpleasant side-effects, although some experience only a few, or find that they disappear after a while. Some side-effects may be eliminated by changing to a different brand, type or dosage of HRT.

The common side effects are:

- breast-soreness
- headaches
- muscle cramps
- fluid retention
- increased blood-pressure
- depression.

- weight-gain
- bloatedness
- nausea
- swollen ankles
- dizziness

Which HRT should I take?

HRT comes in several forms. It can be:

- swallowed as tablets;
- applied to the skin as patches or gel;
- placed under the skin in implants;
- inserted into the vagina as a cream or pessary.

There are many types available and your GP should be able to suggest which he or she thinks is the best for you. It is a good idea to discuss in detail which symptoms are bothering you, as some treatments are better than others for particular problems.

Take note!

Some women who haven't yet reached the menopause are being prescribed low-dose HRT as a way of counteracting some of the effects of drug treatment (more on this in Chapter 5).

'Endometriosis after a hysterectomy'

Once the ovaries have been removed, you would expect to have no more problems with endometriosis. However, some women do still have difficulties. The reasons for this are thought to be that small amounts of the ovary are sometimes left behind, and continue to produce oestrogen; and also because the adrenal glands may still produce sex hormones which can be converted into oestrogen by fatty tissue.

Jane, a 57-year-old retired civil servant, says: 'When I was recovering from my hysterectomy, I was dismayed to find that, as well as the pain of the operation, the original pain was still there. I was immediately given HRT patches but this just made me feel worse. I got terrible headaches. Eventually I got in such a state that I forgot to change the patches, and this actually made the headaches go away and reduced the pain. I told my consultant and eventually he tailor-made an HRT patch for me which included progesterone, and which he said would counteract the effects of the oestrogen.'

Take note!

Many endometriosis sufferers have also complained about being given an HRT implant without their consent, during a hysterectomy. This is certainly not ethical, and your permission should be asked before this is done.

Livial – the new HRT

Livial (generic name tibolone) is the first single substance to combine the actions of the three sex hormones oestrogen, progesterone and testosterone. It is not usually prescribed until a year after the last period, to give the womb-lining time to break down. It doesn't stimulate the endometrium and so regular monthly bleeding on this form of HRT is avoided. It is supposed to be good for several reasons: it improves vaginal and urinary skin-quality, and so makes intercourse less painful; it reduces the loss of bone-density and it has no adverse effects on cholesterol or blood-clotting factors. It is thought to be a good brand to use following a hysterectomy.

Two experiences of HRT

Christine, who is currently taking Livial, says: 'I've been on Livial tablets for ten weeks and have found them an improvement. (I had to wait a year after my hysterectomy before Livial was allowed). My previous HRT preparation contained mostly oestrogen and gave me lot of pain. Livial also protects against heart attacks and bone-density loss, just like the usual HRT. It's easy to take – just one tablet a day from a 28-day pack (like the Pill). It feels as though it's breaking everything down rather than building it up, as with oestrogen. I've had no side-effects apart from a very slight bloatedness to start with and a small amount of bleeding at first. But this has settled down, and I feel mentally much better – not up-and-down like I used to be. I've been told that, when I reach about 50, I can come off it and will be just like any other woman of that age. At last I feel as though I'm on an upward spiral; I'm feeling better every month.'

However, Jennifer has had problems with HRT. She says: 'I had oestradiol implants four months after my hysterectomy. With implants you are given a local anaesthetic first, then they make a small incision in the abdominal wall or thigh and insert the implant (a small pellet). The implant doesn't hurt, but the area is a bit sore afterwards and sometimes I've also needed a couple of stitches.

The implant contained 50 ml of oestradiol but I found it ran out after three months; then I had another one which also ran out after three. So I switched to Premarin tablets (natural oestrogen) which made me feel very sick. I then tried two others, including Progynova which I stopped very quickly because it gave me severe chest-pain. Then I went on to patches, but they didn't stick to my skin very well and they itched a lot. Eventually I went back to implants, but I kept needing higher and higher doses. This made me feel totally exhausted. I also had severe nose-bleeds and couldn't concentrate very well. Eventually I was sent for a blood test which revealed I had dangerously high levels of oestrogen in my blood, so I had to come off HRT immediately. After these experiences, I'd never take HRT again.'

The natural progesterone debate

One school of thought is now suggesting that it is extra progesterone, not oestrogen, that needs to be given during the menopause as, at this time, progesterone production drops to almost nothing whereas small amounts of oestrogen are still made. Most HRT formulas do include synthetic progesterone, but researchers such as American doctor John Lee believe that it is very different from the natural hormone progesterone. He recommends natural progesterone cream to many of his patients, as he believes it can actually restore bone-growth. Some of his patients have reported that their PMS and water retention vanished with progesterone cream.

Many fresh foods contain progesterone-like ingredients. Mexican yam, for instance, contains diosgenin – a substance which needs only one change to become progesterone itself. However, how Mexican yam works in the body is not really known.

A list of doctors prescribing natural progesterone cream is available from the Nutrition Line (see Useful Addresses). You can also obtain wild yam progesterone as a cream, oil, tablet or capsule over the counter at some chemists. The equivalent of 6 g a day is an average dose.

8

Infertility

Infertility and endometriosis

Infertility is an inability to conceive. It is important to remember that women with endometriosis are not sterile; they just sometimes take longer to get pregnant. They are therefore often referred to as 'sub-fertile' rather than infertile. Strictly speaking, you can be diagnosed as sub-fertile if you have failed to conceive after 12 months of regular, unprotected intercourse.

How many women are affected?

Various studies suggest that 30–50 per cent of women with endometriosis are infertile, and that endometriosis is the cause of infertility in 30 per cent of all infertile women. Some researchers take that to mean that there is some link between the two – though the nature of the link is still unknown. But what is known is that infertility becomes more likely as the disease progresses. This is one of the reasons that women should be treated for endometriosis as soon as they are diagnosed. But usually it is only women with severe endometriosis who may have difficulty conceiving as a result of their endometriosis.

How could endometriosis affect my fertility?

As we have said, the reasons aren't really known, but some side-effects of endometriosis may contribute – such as damage to the ovaries and Fallopian tubes caused by the disease, adhesions and scar-tissue resulting from the disease or from surgery, irregular periods and sex (because of the pain) and possibly there are some hormonal factors. The more severe the endometriosis, the more likely it is to cause an infertility problem – but there are still some women with mild endometriosis who suffer from infertility.

Two types of infertility are usually associated with endometriosis (it may help to read Chapter 1 to refresh your mind before considering these):

Endometrial deposits: these may secrete substances which somehow interfere with pregnancy.

Pelvic damage: some women suffering from endometriosis have ovaries distorted by large chocolate cysts; or the finger-like ends of their Fallopian tubes may be distorted by lesions or blocked by adhesions.

Some other theories

Sperm and egg transport

There is a theory that the hormone-like chemicals called prostaglandins (see Chapter 1), which are produced by areas of endometriosis, enter the Fallopian tubes and affect the transport of the sperm and/or the egg in a way which reduces your chances of conceiving.

Ovarian dysfunction

This theory is based on research which shows that some women with endometriosis don't always release an egg during their menstrual cycle. However, it's difficult to say whether this is caused solely by endometriosis, because it can also happen in women who don't have endometriosis.

LUF syndrome

LUF stands for luteinized unruptured follicle syndrome. Some researchers believe that, in some women with endometriosis, ripe eggs sometimes don't hatch from their follicles but instead stay trapped inside. However, other findings suggest that this is no more likely to happen in endometriosis sufferers than in any other women.

Immunology

It is thought that women with endometriosis have some abnormalities in their immune system (see Chapter 2), and that this might play a role in stopping a fertilized egg implanting in the womb – but it's still not clear whether this is the case, so research is continuing.

Prolactin levels

The hormone prolactin is usually secreted during pregnancy, but is sometimes produced outside pregnancy if the pituitary gland grows too big. Too much prolactin is thought to inhibit fertility. Levels are usually checked routinely in women who suffer from sub-fertility, and a drug called bromocriptine is prescribed, which lowers prolactin secretion.

Peritoneal fluid

This fluid is found in the peritoneum (the fluid membrane which lines the abdominal cavity, encasing all the organs). Scavenger-cells are usually present in this fluid to mop up bacteria and endometrial blood, and to stop sperm from swimming out of the Fallopian tubes. Infertile women with endometriosis seem to have a higher number of these scavengers, which could block the movement of the sperm and the egg along the tubes, or even affect the implantation of an embryo.

Recurrent miscarriage

Miscarriage is defined as the failure of pregnancy before week 24, and recurrent miscarriage is if it happens more than twice. After 24 weeks, the loss is termed a stillbirth.

Some early studies show that miscarriage is three times as common in women with endometriosis (mostly within the first 12 weeks of pregnancy). However, other studies indicate that this could have more to do with the woman's previous obstetric history than the presence of endometriosis.

What is the best treatment?

It's important to get treatment for endometriosis as soon as possible because it does sometimes worsen over time. However, because the treatments on offer are only temporary and the disease does usually return, and because all the treatments entail certain risks, women with only mild endometriosis may be advised to follow a wait-and-see approach, i.e. trying for a pregnancy for 6–12 months before embarking on treatment, during which time 20 per cent of women are likely to conceive. After this, drug treatment is usual if the disease has progressed, and then if there are still problems, assisted conception techniques may be suggested.

Take note!

It isn't always a good idea to embark immediately on stressful IVF treatment. The important thing to remember is that lots of women with endometriosis *do* get pregnant. The first things to do are to make sure that you are fit and well, and that your immune system is healthy (advice on this in Chapter 9).

Here are the main treatments for infertility in endometriosis sufferers.

Drug treatment

If the endometriosis deposits aren't too deep, contraceptive pills may at first be suggested as a way of buying time until you feel ready to have a baby or drug treatments such as danazol, progestogens and GnRH analogues (see Chapter 5).

However, there are certain warnings about using these treatments for women who want to conceive, because if you become pregnant while on hormone therapy, there is a chance that the baby may be deformed. So treatment is always started when you are sure you aren't pregnant. Also, some women still ovulate when on the treatment, so it is advisable to use barrier methods of contraception while having drug treatment.

Furthermore, pregnancy shouldn't be attempted until you've had a normal period after stopping treatment, to give the body time to readjust. Progesterone treatment is also not a good option for women considering pregnancy soon, because it can suppress ovulation for quite a while after the treatment has finished – sometimes for up to a year.

How successful is drug treatment?

Pregnancy-rate statistics for endometriosis sufferers following treatment aren't reliable yet, as they are so varied. With the Pill they range from 5 to 75 per cent according to different reports, and there are also some varying statistics with danazol. But what is known is that pregnancy occurs sooner rather than later after treatment, because at that stage you are at your most free from endometriosis. The longer you wait, the more likely it is that endometriosis will reappear.

Surgery

Depending on the degree of endometriosis, reconstruction can be done with a laparotomy or using a laparoscopy and lasers. Endometrial deposits can be cut or burnt away, any adhesions, damaged ovaries or tubes removed, and organs restored to their correct positions. Some reports indicate that laser surgery conserves fertility better because less tissue is destroyed and scar-tissue doesn't result, but there are no reliable figures on this.

Surgery is definitely a good option if you have large cysts or extensive problems which are not easily treatable with drugs. If you are older, you might also feel that you don't have enough time for the wait-and-see approach, or for drug treatment, which takes at least six months.

Disadvantages of surgery

One disadvantage is that surgery might lead to more adhesions, which could contribute further to infertility. It's sometimes thought best to use a combination of surgery and drug treatment, because it's impossible to remove all the sites with surgery alone: the surgeon can't see microscopic patches of endometriosis or treat endometriosis in sensitive areas such as on the organs (see Chapter 6).

How successful is surgery?

With conservative surgery during a laparotomy, the pregnancy rate is 75 per cent in mild cases, 65 per cent in moderate cases and 50 per cent in severe cases. Other reports on success-rates after surgery range from 38 to 87.7 per cent, so the results are somewhat unreliable again. But what is known is that the success afterwards really depends on the extent of the disease before the treatment.

Will the baby be healthy?

Yes – though unfortunately women with endometriosis have a slightly higher rate of miscarriage and ectopic pregnancy (i.e. the foetus develops outside the womb). The higher rate of ectopic pregnancy is probably due to Fallopian tube damage. The danger-signs are a slight bleeding 7–14 days after a missed period, mild soreness or pain getting sharper later, and also fainting and nausea. Help should be sought immediately as it's potentially life-threatening, because it can cause the Fallopian tube to rupture resulting in serious internal bleeding.

Fertility treatments

After your endometriosis has been treated, you may go on to have fertility treatment if you haven't yet fallen pregnant. This may entail the following procedures and tests.

Sex during your fertile stage

A lot of people are unaware that there is a relatively short time each month when a woman can get pregnant. It is only 48 hours after ovulation, i.e. the release of egg. If your cycle is 28 days, this will usually be Day 14 (if Day 1 is the start of your period). But actually there are seven days when you can conceive, because the sperm can survive for about five days inside a woman's body waiting for the egg. So five days before the egg is released and two days after are your most fertile times. Simply buying an ovulation prediction kit, which measures the hormones in urine, may help you fall pregnant.

Keeping temperature charts

In the first instance a woman is often asked to keep a temperature chart because this gives doctors a clue as to whether she is releasing any eggs at all. A woman's central body-temperature usually goes up by a fraction of a degree when she ovulates. However, because you have to take your temperature first thing every day, and record it, this is sometimes thought to put undue stress on some women (an ovulation kit, as mentioned above, might be better).

Undergoing infertility tests

Blood tests: these are usually done on Day 21 of your cycle. They test the levels of the various reproductive hormones in your bloodstream (progesterone is thought to be at its highest when you have ovulated). Your partner may also take a semen test for analysis at the same time.

Post-coital tests: if the blood and semen tests prove inconclusive, you may have a post-coital test whereby mucus from your cervix is sent for analysis after sex. If live, active sperm are seen, then the test is normal.

If there are problems with either of these, further tests may follow:

- ultrasound scan;
- Fallopian tube testing;
- laparoscopy;
- falloscopy (a flexible telescope inserted into the Fallopian tubes to make sure they aren't scarred or blocked or to clear debris from their ends);
- other sperm tests.

For more information on this, and on further, more comprehensive tests which may follow, you can contact one of the charities listed in Useful Addresses, or read one of the books listed under this chapter in Further Reading at the back of the book.

Taking fertility drugs

Your doctor may suggest taking a fertility drug like Clomid (Clomid and Serophene are both trade-names for clomiphene citrate). This drug is used to treat ovulation failure, and works by simulating the ovaries into producing several mature eggs at the same time.

Using assisted conception techniques

What is IVF?

IVF stands for *in vitro* fertilization. It is normally used in conjunction with a fertility drug like Clomid. The patient is then monitored with ultrasound equipment to find out when one of the ovary sacs will burst open. As the time approaches, a fine needle is passed through the wall of abdomen to suck out some of these ripe eggs, which are then mixed with the partner's sperm. Once fertilization has taken place, they may be put directly into womb at some stage.

> Helen, a 35-year-old accountant, started IVF after a laparoscopy revealed she had mild endo which could be interfering with one of her Fallopian tubes.
>
> 'I was put on Zoladex first of all, for six months, which sometimes gave me terrible hot flushes and quite painful breasts, but which seemed to make my usual PMS symptoms disappear completely. Then I was told I could have IVF treatment immediately, or wait three months and then try. The consultant explained that, during my laparoscopy, they had

flushed out my Fallopian tubes and I might want to see whether that had worked first of all.

But I decided to go for IVF straight away. First of all, my husband and I went for basic tests – such as a scan to check that my ovaries were working properly and a Day 21 progesterone blood test to make sure that my hormones were working properly too. Also I had a vaginal swab taken to rule out infections such as PID.

Then I was given the nasal spray buserelin, which I had to take every four hours. Apparently, if you take this drug first, your ovaries are more likely to respond to the fertility drugs. I found it horrendous trying to remember it all the time and had to carry a little alarm clock around with me. I was quite worried because they said that, if I took it just ten minutes late, it would mean that my female hormone levels would go back up.

They then scanned me to see whether my ovaries were in a sufficiently menopausal state to start taking fertility drugs. I started on the Pergonol injections (a fertility drug) on a Friday, and was given an injection every day and scanned each day to see how my eggs were developing. They have to be careful not to over-stimulate you, because this can be dangerous.

The following Friday, they looked to see whether I'd produced enough eggs for them to operate – which I had. Then, ten days later, I was taken into the operating theatre, the eggs were extracted and then fertilized with my husband's sperm in a test-tube. Two days later I went back again, and the eggs were inserted into me very simply via a catheter (it's just like having a smear). Then we had to wait for two weeks to see if I was pregnant.

I had this procedure done twice unsuccessfully, but then I started going to stress management classes, run by my hospital for women with fertility problems. I learned how to breathe properly and to do self-hypnosis and was encouraged to talk about any worries which might be blocking me from becoming pregnant. For instance, I realized that I was very anxious about money problems should I become pregnant, although I didn't really need to be. Within three months (in between IVF attempts) I got pregnant naturally. Now I'm about to give birth. I can't tell what helped me conceive – all I can say is that I'm delighted!'

What is GIFT?

GIFT stands for Gamete Intra-Fallopian Transfer, and means that the gametes (the sperm and egg) are put back into the womb at an earlier stage than in ordinary IVF treatment. They are usually flushed into the Fallopian tubes where fertilization may be more likely to take place because of the more natural environment.

Is there any alternative treatment?

Vitamin E, zinc and the herbal extract *vitex agnus castus* are said to improve fertility; treatments such as acupuncture for the pain, chiropractice and homeopathy have also been found to be beneficial. Nutrition and exercise may also help. For instance, a high-protein diet and B vitamins are thought to be especially important (see Chapter 9).

Should I keep trying?

Paula says, 'When I was told that I had virtually no chance of conceiving because of endometriosis and because my husband's sperm-count was low, we decided we didn't really mind not being able to have children. We both have fulfilling careers and we didn't want to go through the trauma of IVF. After a course of danazol, we stopped using contraceptives, but within two years I was surprised and delighted to find I was pregnant. We were advised after that to try quickly again if we wanted any more children, and just sixteen months later our next one came along. So I can't help thinking if you're relaxed about pregnancy it is more likely to happen.'

Joanne's experiences were very different: 'I've decided that, although I'm only 27, I'd like to have a hysterectomy. Trying to have a baby has made me feel suicidal. I just can't cope with my hopes constantly being dashed. Between us, my husband and I have decided that my quality of life and us being happy together is more important than a baby. I want to put it all behind me and get on with my life. And I realize, too, that now the pressure is off I wasn't quite as bothered about it as I thought I was. Talking about it in the endometriosis support groups has really helped me come to this decision.'

Is pregnancy a cure for endometriosis?

Doctors have long believed that pregnancy is a cure for endometriosis. It is true in so far as pregnancy can help endometrial deposits to clear up because your periods stop for nine months. However, although many women do report a lessening of their symptoms during pregnancy, they do often say it returns afterwards – and the more severe the case is, the more severely it usually returns.

But if you feel better during pregnancy, a way to lengthen the time of remission is to breast-feed, as ovulation is believed to be suppressed by breast-feeding. You can read literature from the National Childbirth Trust (see Useful Addresses) to find out the best way to do this.

However, there have been some reports to the American Endometriosis

Association of the disease worsening during pregnancy, although no studies have yet been done on this.

Having said that, even if you want to take your chances and see if it works for you, you should still carefully weigh up whether you do want a baby at this point in your life.

Pointers to consider

1 Don't rush into it.
2 Talk to women from your local endometriosis group who are in a similar situation.
3 Speak to a counsellor sensitive to your situation, to help you sort out your feeling about this.

9
Coping Strategies

Coping with your pain

Learning to cope with the pain is important for endometriosis sufferers. Here are some practical tips on things which have helped other sufferers (in alphabetical order).

Baths and relaxation

Many women find that encouraging muscles to relax, either through taking a bath or practising relaxation, can help period pain considerably. Breathing deeply may also help.

Diet

Eating a sufficient, varied and good diet is particularly important during a period. Many women have also found reducing salt (which aggravates PMS bloating), sugar (which can cause yeast problems), alcohol and caffeine intake (which make you feel more irritable and stressed), beneficial during their period. (There is more about diet later in this chapter.)

Exercise

Exercise is one of the best measures for combating pain, as it results in the body producing its own natural painkillers. Cycling, swimming and fast walking are particularly useful. Exercise can also be helpful if only to take your mind off your pain for a few seconds.

If you find that even walking is too painful, you could try the following exercise instead:

1 Lie flat on floor with a pillow behind your knees.
2 Start from the bottom and work up, tensing your feet, calves, thighs, buttocks, etc., right up to your neck and facial muscles.
3 Hold each set of muscles tight for 5–10 seconds, then let your breath out. It should take only about ten minutes in all, but you should notice a result!

(There is more on exercise later in this chapter.)

Flotation therapy

Flotation therapy is reported to be good for pain relief. You literally float on the top of a tank of water, which contains a salt solution to stop you sinking. It is also thought that the experience of floating alters the electrical activity in the brain, promoting profound relaxation.

Heat and cold

Heat-pads or hot-water bottles can reduce muscle spasms and increase the flow of blood. Also a sauna or warm bath can have the same effect. Likewise, rubbing something cold – such as packet of frozen peas – on the site of the pain until the skin feels numb, can reduce pain.

Keeping a pain diary or scrapbook

Many sufferers have found it useful to keep a simple diary of their pain, to help to take their mind off it and as a useful resource to show their GP or consultant.

Christine says: 'Keeping a diary helped me to put my frustrations down on paper, and then to let go of them. I also showed it to my GP who said it was great help to him to see cyclical pattern.'

Elizabeth found that it helped to create a scrapbook: 'I got the idea from one of the self-help books,' she says. 'I'm not an arty person but I got a scrapbook and some glue and crayons. I stuck in my favourite quotes from books I'd found useful, cartoons from the paper, a photo of myself and some information on drugs which my doctor had given me, and also vitamins I was taking. That particular self-help book also encouraged me to try and picture what my pain looks like and even draw it. It was very hard at first but there is no right or wrong way of doing it. My drawings of coloured blobs on scraps of paper (often done in five minutes at work) won't win any prizes, but they gave me a sort of physical map of how I felt at that moment and this was very useful.

I also write down how I feel in my special book and give my pain a star rating. Five stars is the worst – that's when I find it hard just to put my socks on in the morning. The scrapbook has really help me continue working when I've been in great pain.'

Massage

Massage can also be very helpful in coping with pain. Massage involves a variety of rubbing and kneading techniques which help to relieve tension, improve circulation and reduce pain and high blood-pressure. You could see a qualified practitioner, or you could try the following self-help techniques yourself:

- For period pain: using a V-stroke from one hip-bone down to the pubic hairline and up to the other hip-bone, firmly apply your fingertips in a circular direction just above the pubic hairline.
- For ovulation pain: apply massage in a circular motion just below the inside ankle-bone.
- For back-pain: massage the bottom of your foot along the inside arch.

Orgasm

Orgasm can be good for period pain as it naturally causes the womb to contract and helps to expel blood; it can also help congestive symptoms.

Painkillers (see Chapter 5)

Pain Management

There are hundreds of pain-management centres in the UK to which your doctor can refer you – such as the one run by St Thomas' Hospital in London – as well as private charitable organizations, such as Painwise UK, Pain Concern UK or UNWIND (see Useful Addresses at the back of the book).

Ten tips on coping with pain

Jan Sadler, a member of Painwise UK, gives the following advice on how to cope with a flare-up:

1 Keep positive: the most important thing is actually to decide to take charge of the situation by facing and accepting it. Accept that it has happened and there is nothing to be gained by blaming anyone, especially yourself. A really helpful phrase to say to yourself is, 'Be still – this will pass'.
2 Plan: try not to let yourself get so overwhelmed that you abandon all the helpful strategies you have learned in the past. Write a list, and mentally decide which technique you need at the moment.
3 Relax: at least once a day make space for 15–20 minutes of deep relaxation. Find a quiet place and use whatever method suits you. One of the simplest methods employed in meditation is to 'watch' your breath as it goes in and out, and as your mind wanders gently bring it back to your breath again.
4 Use affirmations: this is simply repeating a few special words which reflect how you would like to be, such as 'I am peaceful and calm'. Make up some useful ones which you can write on little cards to refer to when you need them.
5 Visualization: spend some time creating pictures in your mind. Imagine

yourself floating in a balloon or imagine changing your pain into something more comfortable, e.g. burning pains could be cooled by standing under a waterfall.

6 Pace yourself: cut down your sitting, standing and walking times to a level you can cope with – even if it's only half a minute at a time. Then get a timer and start a pacing programme. Set your timer to the number of minutes you've decided to spend on each activity, and when it rings change tasks. Very slowly increase these times.

7 Keep your body active: exercise is very important, even it you're just starting with stretching your fingers and toes. Just make a start and then space the exercises out throughout the day. Swimming is particularly good as the water is supportive, preventing the dragging pain you may feel when walking.

8 Keep your mind active: try to keep to your daily routine as much as possible. Even if it's just reading a book or watching TV, it can help distract you.

9 Use helping aids: try some of the other pain relief methods mentioned in this book, such as a TENS machine, aromatherapy or acupuncture.

10 Be patient: that means living here and now, but not with one foot planted in next week. In yearning for the future the whole time, we miss everything around us and simply create more tension for ourselves. Be kind to yourself and focus on what you can do this moment and not what you can't!

More information is in Jan Sadler's book, *Natural Pain Relief*, listed in Further Reading.

Pelvic exercises

Congestion before periods can be relieved by pelvic exercises which tone up the pelvic-floor muscles, stimulate circulation in the area and help drain away any excess fluid.

To find out which are your pelvic muscles try stopping the urine flow when you next go to the loo – the ones you naturally find yourself using are your pelvic floor muscles. If you can stop the flow instantly, your muscles are in good shape. But if you can't, you may like to try the following exercise:

- Lie flat on your back with your knees bent and your feet flat on floor.
- Imagine pulling something in and up into your vagina. You'll probably find yourself tightening your buttocks as you do this, but try to make sure it isn't only them you're tightening.
- Hold the muscles for a slow count of five and then release them.

- You could test how well you are doing by holding your fingers in your vagina and trying to tighten the pelvic muscles around them.

There are also several books giving advice on pelvic exercises (all of which are unfortunately out of print but may be available at your library): *Lifting the Curse*, by B. Kingston and *Painless Periods*, by M. Storch and C. Carmichael.

TENS

TENS stands for transcutaneous electrical nerve stimulation. This method of pain-relief involves using a tiny electronic device, smaller than a Walkman, which has two to four electrodes attached to it. These are placed on the body in the area of the pain, and then the machine is switched on, generating a tiny electrical impulse through the body. They can be used with good effects for anything from half-an-hour to eight hours a day. They work by stimulating endorphins in the body, which are our own natural painkillers.

You could ask your GP or local hospital pain clinic if they will lend you one. Otherwise you can buy one from RDG Medical (0181 660 4374) or Spembly Medical (0800 515413). Prices range from £58 to £115.

Coping with your feelings

Depression

A lot of women with endometriosis are also depressed – 63 per cent reported depression as a symptom of endometriosis in the 1984 NES survey. As we've said already, it is hardly surprising that women suffering from endometriosis feel depressed when they are dealing with such a confusing, debilitating and little-understood illness. Women suffering from endometriosis often say the following things about endometriosis:

- 'No one believes me!'
- 'My friends don't understand why I'm in pain!'
- 'Everyone thinks I'm a hypochondriac!'

If you feel like this, you might ask your GP to refer you to a counsellor, so that you can at least get a sympathetic ear. But apart from endometriosis, there might be other reasons why you feel depressed – things that need sorting out. But the main thing to remember is: **you're not going mad!**

Jackie says: 'I've had a few appointments with my practice counsellor – really just to vent the ghost of the way I've been treated in the past year.

I'd felt very angry that my continued pain was ignored, and that at one stage I was even sent to a psychiatrist because of it. I felt it was important to get over this – almost to right the medical wrong. I then discussed my thoughts about the future, such as about my fertility and my relationship with my boyfriend. I've found it helpful as it has put things into perspective. It was also good to have someone acknowledging my feelings without blaming me for feeling the way I did.'

Your partner and family

During a seminar on pain management, run for the NES by an organization called Painwise UK, it became clear that one of the biggest problems for endometriosis sufferers was the guilt they felt about their partners and families. Sufferers often felt that, because of the pain, they weren't able to be proper mothers or wives.

If you are in this situation, you might find it helpful to take your husband to a mixed session at your local endometriosis group. Alternatively you could get your partner or other members of your family to read some of the literature on the subject, so that they will understand exactly what you're going through.

Eleanor's partner Nick says: 'When I knew more about the condition it helped me to be more understanding. I could see why Eleanor was so frustrated by the lack of correct diagnosis. It also made me realize that it was good for her to talk about it, as in the past she had suffered a lot in silence.'

Jackie describes some of the difficulties endometriosis has caused in her relationship: 'I met my partner just over two years ago, and it has been a relationship of discovery for both of us. The endometriosis has made me – and consequently us – address issues a lot earlier than you would normally have to. For instance, we've had to address the problem of painful sex – and it's been quite difficult working out whether I'm tensing up because of the anticipated pain or whether sex is just painful in itself.

Endometriosis can also be a difficult concept to put across – what it means, how it feels, the pain, the surgery and the drug treatments. But quite early on in our relationship I was quite open about it, referring to endometriosis as a ''WYSIWYG'' – i.e. what you see is what you get. If I felt dreadful, I couldn't lie about it or pretend the pain didn't exist and would acknowledge it as a not-so-good day.

But fortunately my partner is loving and caring enough for endometriosis not to be a 'problem'. At times, I admit, I would test him to see how much my having endometriosis affected us – but he would just say that he couldn't separate the two, or that me not having endometriosis wouldn't necessarily make us any better, however much he wished I didn't have the pain; that this thing unfortunately is part of me, and he thinks I'm strong enough to handle it, and that he loves me as a whole (this is beginning to sound like a Mills & Boon romance, isn't it!).

However, being in a relationship brings with it a new set of issues: where do we go from here, can I conceive, do I want to conceive, do I want to conceive in this relationship, how much time do I have? How much time do I have between treatments? All those sorts of things!'

Coping with problems about sex

Lack of sex is a great problem in the relationships of endometriosis sufferers. The NES survey (as we saw in Chapter 4) reported that 55 per cent of sufferers experience painful sex. This can cause great strain between you and your partner, who may understandably feel very rejected. Talking is always the best option, or you may even consider going to RELATE if this is difficult.

Tips on how to make sex less painful

- Make sure you are fully aroused before penetration: it is less likely to cause pain, because you are then properly lubricated. Full arousal also causes the vagina to elongate and the cervix to move further up and so you are less likely to bash sensitive areas, such as the Pouch of Douglas or the pelvic organs. It also makes it less likely that your vagina muscles will close spontaneously.
- If you have problems with a dry vagina (one of the menopausal symptoms which can result from drug treatment), try a lubricant such as KY jelly, Replens vaginal moisturiser or vitamin E oil rubbed into the vagina.
- Also bear in mind that, just because you don't have penetration, it doesn't mean you're not having sex! You could try arousing each other in different ways and experimenting with other types of sex. A self-help manual may give you some ideas!

Take note: Pain with deep penetration during intercourse, or painful contractions during orgasm, can sometimes be result of the uterine muscles becoming sensitive during drug treatment.

What does RELATE DO?

Many women experience relationship problems when they suffer from endometriosis. Not only are they in pain, stressed and tired, often they can only just about hold down a job, and on top of that may (as we have already said) find sexual intercourse a problem. So again it's hardly surprising that there might be greater strains in a relationship.

RELATE provides general relationship counselling, but can also refer people for sex therapy. Counsellors aren't paid, but RELATE usually asks for a contribution towards their overheads (such as the cost of training and the building rental) – though they never turn anyone away because of lack of funds. Contact your local RELATE office (listed in the phone book) or the head office (in Useful Addresses).

After being treated for endometriosis and giving birth to their first child, Cheryl used a particular sex therapy called 'sensate focus' to help re-establish a sexual relationship with her husband.

She recalls: 'We were told to start by spending a week kissing and cuddling each other for twenty minutes a day. We weren't allowed to touch genital areas and my breasts were also out of bounds. So this felt very safe, as I knew it wouldn't lead to sex. It felt great, like we were getting each other back after a long time apart.

Two weeks later we moved on to the next stage: massage. Again, sexual areas of the body were out of bounds. And we were instructed to tell each other about the kind of touch we liked and disliked. I don't like any kind of light, feathery touch which feels like it tickles, and at first I had trouble explaining to Paul that I wanted him to be firm but not too heavy-handed. But eventually he got it down to a fine art.

The following week we were allowed to touch each other's genital areas – but not masturbate them. We were, however, allowed to take it in turns to masturbate ourselves while the other looked on.

This worked so well that we found it difficult to hold back from going further. And the next week, when we were still not allowed to have intercourse, we couldn't stop ourselves from steaming ahead.

We turned up at the doctor's surgery giggling like two naughty school kids. He took one look at us and said, ''Get out of here! You don't need me any more''. But he added that we knew where to find him if we had trouble again. Six years on we're still OK – although Paul sometimes says he wishes we had sex more often . . . but at least we talk about these things now.'

What does counselling do?

There are many different types of counselling available in Britain today. Some involve in-depth psycho-analysis which could go on for several years; others are short-term and very goal-orientated – i.e. you come with a view to solving a very specific problem. All will help you explore your feelings about your illness and how it affects your relationships. But they won't tell you what to do – their purpose is really to help you understand yourself better.

The thing to remember is that counselling is a positive step. More and more people seek counselling these days, and it certainly doesn't mean you are going mad.

You can apply to have counselling on the NHS through your doctor or else you could go to a private therapist who charge anything upwards from £15 (most will operate a sliding scale according to your means).

For more information contact the British Association of Counselling (see Useful Addresses) or read *The Counselling Handbook*, by Susan Quilliam and Ian Grove-Stephensen (see Further Reading).

Jane says: 'I saw a counsellor at the college where I was a mature student. Although she wasn't as empathetic and warm as I'd hoped, she did help me come to terms with the anger I felt towards doctors. Having been misdiagnosed for 40 years and made to feel like a malingerer, I was understandably very upset. She helped me to be able to talk to doctors in a level voice, and to see that my anger against them was destructive for me. Sometimes, when I'd finished a session, I went away feeling I could put all those worries down and for a moment it was as though I was walking on air!'

Self-help groups

Time and time again, endometriosis sufferers have said how much support groups have helped them. There are over 38 local groups run by the National Endometriosis Society (NES – see Useful Addresses), which also runs a telephone help-line. The groups do all sorts of things, from sharing their feelings, to advice on relaxation techniques – and have sessions which include partners. Some find it helpful in practical ways; others say that just sharing their feelings makes them feel less isolated. If there isn't an endometriosis group in your area, you could try joining a general women's self-help group.

Janet says: 'When I first went to the endometriosis support group I just cried and cried. Then they helped me write a letter to my consultant putting down my experiences clearly and simply. The letter helped me get a proper consultation with him and to be at last taken seriously. Also the group helped me to fight to get my early retirement entitlement. It took 18 months, and in the end I had to settle on arthritis as the cause, even though it was endometriosis. But their support still helped me not to give up and settle for less.'

Dietary advice

It is generally assumed that a basic healthy diet is good for endometriosis sufferers. The 'rules' are simple:

- eat plenty of vegetables and fresh fruit;
- eat as many wholefoods as possible, such as wholegrain cereals;
- where possible, grill, steam or stew foods rather than fry them;
- eat more foods rich in essential fatty acids, such as seeds, nuts and grains;
- cook in oil rather than fat;
- eat low-fat versions of dairy products (e.g. skimmed milk);
- cut down on sugar;
- reduce your intake of salt and animal fats;
- choose white meats, such as chicken, rather than red meat;
- drink less coffee, tea and fizzy drinks;
- drink at least six glasses of water a day.

Don't expect to change your diet overnight. Try out new ideas as you go along and transform your eating habits gradually – you might even find it quite exciting!

Vitamin and mineral supplements

Some women have noticed an improvement in general health when just taking an ordinary multi-vitamin and mineral tablet. If you don't want the hassle of taking a lot of different tablets, you could try taking one for a few months to see if it improves your symptoms. Different brands vary considerably, so if you react negatively to one brand, try another.

Alternatively, if you would like to go into it in more detail the NES advises seeking an alternative practitioner who specializes in nutritional or vitamin therapies. You could find one by contacting the Society for the Promotion of Nutritional Therapy (SPNT), the Institute of Optimum Nutrition, or the Women's Nutritional Advisory Service (see Useful Addresses).

Evening Primrose oil

Suggested daily intake: 2–3 500 mg tablets for general health; 4–6 500 mg tablets for PMS

Evening Primrose oil (brand-names include Efamol – large pharmaceutical chains now make their own brands) is thought to be good for alleviating PMS, and can also reduce the side-effects of drug treatment (such as the tiredness and water retention caused by danazol). This oil contains a substance called GLA (gamma linoleic acid), thought to enhance the production of a particular prostaglandin, which regulates several of the body-functions involved in PMS.

Natural sources of GLA include cold-pressed safflower oil (available from health food shops). Starflower oil (sometimes called borage oil) is thought to contain three times as much GLA as Evening Primrose oil, but in a somewhat different chemical form. Further research is needed to assess its potential.

> Suzanne, who had a cyst removed from her right ovary, says: 'Primrose oil has definitely eased my pain a great deal. I find if I just stop it for one day I begin to get pains down the back of my legs.'

Dolomite (calcium/magnesium)

Daily intake: 200–800 mg.

Calcium and magnesium improve muscle-tone, making the contractions during your period more even and less painful. Calcium absorption may be reduced if your magnesium intake is too low, and so they are usually taken together. For still better absorption, take calcium with low doses of vitamins D and E. Vitamin E improves the healing of scar-tissue caused by internal endometrial bleeding. However, as dolomite is not absorbed easily, other sources of calcium and magnesium may be better.

Magnesium sources: green, leafy vegetables, grapefruit, figs, apples, nuts and seeds.

Calcium sources: dried beans, green vegetables, peanuts, walnuts, sunflower seeds, sardines.

Vitamin B6 (Pyridoxine)

Suggested daily intake: 100 mg (50 mg twice a day), together with 25–50 mg of vitamin B complex (depending on the strength).

Vitamin B6 reduces symptoms of PMS, such as depression, bloatedness, headache and breast tenderness. It seems particularly to help endometriosis sufferers who experience these symptoms for the whole of the month. It is a good idea to take it with vitamin B complex for a balanced intake. (Be careful not to overdose on B vitamins as it can lead to nerve damage.)

Vitamin B6 also helps with the side-effects of such hormone treatments as danazol, duphaston and Primolut-N – especially the tiredness and depression they can cause.

Natural sources: brewer's yeast (avoid this if you're sensitive to yeast), wheatgerm, cabbage, eggs.

Vitamin E

Daily intake: from 200–600 international units (iu) to be increased gradually.

Vitamin E is important for endometriosis sufferers because it keeps scar-tissue soft and flexible, reducing the pain caused by adhesions. It is best to start with 100 iu twice daily and to increase gradually (be extra gradual in your increase if you have blood-pressure problems).

Take note: anyone with high blood-pressure should not exceed 400 iu. daily without medical supervision. Anyone on anticoagulant therapy should also avoid it without careful medical supervision.

Natural sources: green vegetables, wholegrain cereal, soya beans and eggs.

Vitamin C

Daily intake: 500 mg to 1 g.

Extra vitamin C can help if you suffer from heavy bleeding, as it strengthens blood-vessel walls and aids the absorption of iron (which helps make red blood-cells). It can also help you heal after surgery, and some endometriosis sufferers have reported that it is good for pain. It also helps strengthen the immune system, helping you to fight colds and infections better.

Natural sources: green vegetables, potatoes, citrus fruits, blackcurrants.

Vitamin D

Daily intake: 350–400 iu.

Vitamin D is important for calcium absorption and helps bone formation, so it may be useful in preventing osteoporosis.

Natural sources: fatty fish, eggs.

Selenium

Daily intake: 200 mcg.

Selenium is a trace element, which is taken together with vitamins A, C and E. It is available in several forms, some of which have a yeast base which is thought to improve the absorption of selenium. (If you have yeast or candida problems, check the label to make sure you buy one without yeast.) Selenium and vitamin E are supposed to give protection to the body, producing an anti-inflammatory type of effect. Selenium is also known to strengthen the immune system which, as we know, is an important factor in fighting endometriosis. Vitamin E is also known to reduce adhesions and is also used to treat arthritis.

Natural sources: garlic, broccoli, tomatoes, wheatgerm, tuna.

Zinc

Daily intake: 10–30 mg.

Zinc is another mineral thought to help in the treatment of PMS by countering depression; it also promotes healing and fertility.

Natural sources: eggs, oysters, herring, wheatgerm, seeds, nuts.

Supplement Dos and Don'ts

- Don't take isolated vitamins or minerals without the advice of a qualified practitioner.
- Generally take supplements with meals, because then they are more easily absorbed. However, there are some exceptions, such as zinc which is thought to be absorbed better at night on an empty stomach.
- When buying a multi-vitamin supplement, opt for one with a wide and balanced variety of minerals and vitamins.
- Don't be tempted to take supplements instead of balanced meals.

More Specific Diet Guidelines

Some sufferers have found the following specific dietary treatments helpful.

The Natural Oestrogen Diet

Some researchers believe that, by eating foods containing weak plant oestrogens (isoflavonoids), you may actually be able to reduce the amount of oestrogen in your own body. However, the idea is very controversial and the benefits haven't yet been fully substantiated.

Foods which are a rich source of these include:

- dried fruits
- cabbages and turnips
- berries, peas and pulses
- beans, nuts and seeds
- unrefined grain-products, such as rye products
- soya products such as tofu.

It isn't advisable to change your diet radically without detailed advice and supervision.

Extra vitamins C, E and Betacarotene

A diet rich in vitamins C, E and betacarotene is thought to reduce cell damage and the growth of tumours in your body by interfering with the body's metabolic reactions. You could take vitamin supplements which include these, or just increase foods containing these vitamins.

Vitamin C: blackcurrants and other fruits, peppers, potatoes and green vegetables.

Vitamin E: eggs, butter, seeds, nuts, oily fish.

Betacarotene: spinach, carrots, tomatoes, peaches.

The high-fibre diet

A high fibre diet is thought to reduce the levels of oestrogen in your body, because it prevents excreted oestrogen being reabsorbed in the bowel. This sort of diet is also good for constipation and bowel problems. However, a very high-fibre diet can interfere with the absorption of nutrients and worsen irritable bowel syndrome.

You could increase your fibre intake by eating more:

- wholemeal bread (it contains twice as much fibre as white bread);
- fruit – a soluble fibre which inhibits the effects of cholesterol;
- vegetables such as peas, beans, lentils, leaf and root vegetables, and salads;
- breakfast cereals made with wholewheat or grains, wholewheat pasta, brown rice, oats and rye bread.

The macrobiotic diet

The macrobiotic diet is based on eating whole, unrefined foods, such as bread, cereals, grains, pasta, vegetables, fruits, seeds, beans, certain fish and seafoods including seaweed. No refined sugar, dairy products or meat (butter, sugar, eggs, ham and beef are thought to be particularly bad) are included. A macrobiotic diet is all about getting back to basics, i.e. natural, organic food without chemicals which might interfere with the natural processes of the body.

For more information contact The Institute for Complementary Medicine listed in the Useful Addresses section at back of book. The Community Health Foundation also runs macrobiotic cookery courses.

The anti-candida diet

Candida is quite a problem for many endometriosis sufferers, and can be combated by a yeast-free, sugar-free diet, designed to stop the growth of the yeast-like organism in the body called *candida albicans*.

Candida albicans lives in the urethra and alimentary canal (the passage from the mouth to the anus) of all human beings, and also in the vagina. It is like the infection which occurs in similar areas, called thrush. Your body naturally keeps candida in check, but when your immune system is weakened the fungus can multiply and spread.

Certain conditions – such as smoking too much, being over-stressed, suffering from deficiencies in vitamin B6 and C and zinc, using oral corticosteroids long-term, or taking antibiotics for long periods of time – are thought to predispose people to candida. Also, certain symptoms such as cravings for sweet foods, bloating and recurrent thrush are supposed to be indicative of *candida albicans*. Some researchers even believe that candida can get into your bloodstream, upsetting the whole body-system. If the immune system is severely disrupted very serious effects can develop which may need urgent medical treatment.

For less serious cases you can get treatment from a nutritional or allergy specialist who may prescribe you anti-fungal remedies and certain vitamins and minerals to strengthen your immune system, as well as putting you on a yeast-free diet. Treatment usually lasts one to six months, depending on how bad it is. (Contact the Institute for Complementary Medicine, listed in Useful Addresses, for a practitioner.)

Food allergies

Allergies can make endometriosis sufferers feel even worse. Some people have found that trying out an elimination diet under the guidance of a qualified therapist can be helpful. The idea is to cut out one type of food at a time – such as wheat, dairy products, meat or whatever – to see if it relieves your symptoms, and then gradually to reintroduce them again.

Angela, who has suffered from severe endometriosis involving the bladder and the intestines, says: 'As well as following a healthy diet, I try to avoid wheat and dairy products which I've discovered result in bloating and cause me more endometriosis pain. Just eating a bit of chocolate can give me a whole weekend of pain!'

For more information on therapists, contact the Institute for Complementary Medicine listed under Useful Addresses.

Changing your lifestyle

The following options may also be of general help to endometriosis sufferers

Losing weight

If you lose *excess* weight, you produce less oestrogen, because fat cells produce small amounts of a weaker form of oestrogen. This rarely matters for younger women, as their usual oestrogen is much greater than the small amounts from fat. However, it does become important at or near the menopause.

Tips on losing weight

There are plenty of books and articles on sensible dieting – you could try *The Food Trap* by Paulette Maisner and Rosemary Turner (see Further Reading). If you think there may be emotional reasons why you find it difficult to lose weight you could try contacting the Eating Disorders Association (see Useful Addresses) who may be able to refer you to a counsellor.

Stopping smoking

Smoking depletes the levels of vitamin B6 and other B vitamins plus vitamin C in the body, which are needed to counteract many of the symptoms of PMS. Women taking HRT will also get less benefit from it if they smoke, and will therefore get less protection against osteoporosis.

If you want to give up smoking, contact the free information and advice service Quitline on: 0800 002200 – or try reading a book (e.g. *The Easy Way to Stop Smoking*, by Allen Carr).

Cutting down on alcohol

Alcohol contains high levels of sugar and can contribute to mood swings. It also acts as a depressant on the nervous system, and so doesn't help when fighting endometriosis. Your GP's surgery has information about safe amounts (two to three units a day) – and what this actually means.

Some sufferers develop alcohol problems, finding it the only way to blot out the pain. For more confidential help, contact Alcohol Concern or your local Alcoholics Anonymous (listed in the phone book).

Stress

Stress could contribute to endometriosis. Not only is it harder to fight an illness if you are under severe stress, but stress can also depress the immune system – and endometriosis is thought to be partly caused by a deficiency in the immune system. It is also thought that, the more stressed you are, the more sharply you experience pain.

Tips on stress-management

1 Write down lists of what you need to do each day and prioritize the tasks.
2 Don't do something just because it's expected of you – learn to say no.
3 If you have a problem, talk about it. If you can't talk to a friend or relative, try counselling (see Chapter 9).
4 Give yourself breaks throughout the day to do something you enjoy – like walking, reading or having a bath.

5 Try to hang on to your sense of humour as much as possible.
6 Avoid making too many life-changes at once.
7 Try not to brood over situations over which you have no control – and try not to hang on to the past.
8 Cultivate a social life.
9 Exercise regularly to reduce tension.
10 Learn to relax. You may want to learn a regular relaxation technique such as breathing exercises, yoga or massage (more on this in Chapter 10).
11 Ask your GP about stress-management courses (see Chapter 10).

Exercise

Exercise is good for you: it keeps your body healthy and improves your circulation. Not only that, vigorous exercise (i.e. exercise which gets you hot and sweaty) produces endorphins – your body's natural painkillers, which make you feel more relaxed and happy.

More specifically, exercise has also been shown more specifically to help with menopausal symptoms such as mood swings, osteoporosis, constipation and other symptoms which might be shared by endometriosis sufferers. Exercise helps to keep any adhesions flexible, and might play a role in keeping your hormonal levels normal. It's also been shown to counteract many of the side-effects of danazol.

Angela, who has severe endometriosis, says: 'I try to swim two or three times a week. If I miss a session I really notice it.'

Jacqueline says: 'I felt much better when I did two or three exercise classes a week. I think, as well as making me more relaxed and better able to fight the pain, it made me feel more positive. When one class stopped and I began to stop going, my pain definitely got worse.'

Tranquillizers

Tranquillizers, sleeping pills and antidepressants are often prescribed for chronic pain. But really they should only be used in the short term, because prolonged use of certain drugs (such as the benzodiazepines like Valium and Mogadon) can be addictive. They can also sometimes make the pain worse, interfere with your sleep patterns and can contribute to depression. If you have a problem with addiction you can get advice from your doctor on how to withdraw from them slowly, or you could contact the Council for Involuntary Tranquillizer Addiction (see Useful Addresses).

10

Complementary Therapies

Alternative or complementary treatments aim to treat the whole person rather than their disease. For a lot of people, just getting that detailed one-to-one attention offered by complementary therapists – which unfortunately most of our own doctors are unable to give us – can be very therapeutic. But, just as with conventional treatments, it depends on your individual situation and your symptoms as to which will be the best for you. Here (in alphabetical order) are some treatments which other endometriosis sufferers have found helpful.

Acupuncture

Acupuncture is based on the theory that our health is governed by a flow of energy around the body (known as Chi) which travels from one organ to another. A blockage or imbalance in this flow is thought to bring about ill-health.

After taking a detailed history from you, including information about your emotional state as well as your symptoms, the acupuncturist usually attempts to 'unblock' these areas by putting needles into your body at specific points. But don't worry – the needles are much finer than those used for injections, and the patient only feels a light prick as the needle goes through the skin.

Researchers now believe that one of the ways acupuncture works is by creating local anaesthesia, by causing the release of endorphins – a natural painkiller produced by the body.

Acupuncture has been known to help all sorts of gynaecological problems, including painful periods, menopausal symptoms and PMS – though the NES has had mixed reports from endometriosis sufferers about its effectiveness. Some women have found it beneficial, whereas others said that it made their symptoms worse. Some people believe that the traditional method of acupuncture may be more helpful than modern techniques.

For more information on all types of acupuncture contact the British Acupuncture Council, Park House, 206 Latimer Road, London W10 6RE (0181 964 0222).

'I had acupuncture'

Elizabeth, a 34-year-old personal assistant who suffers from endometriosis of the round ligament of the womb, says: 'Acupuncture definitely helped me, as I felt that my immune system was really affected by what was going on in my body. Acupuncture also helps greatly in relieving pain.

I like the fact that the acupuncturist treats you as a whole person, looking at your emotional as well as physical side. When I first went to the acupuncturist she took my pulse and looked at my tongue, which helped her decide which range of points to put the needles in.

But I feel it isn't just the treatment which helps – it's having someone with the space to listen to me. It helps so much just to hear someone say to you, ''I know you're in pain'', and to feel their support.'

Aromatherapy

Aromatherapy uses essential oils, derived from plants and trees, for healing purposes. About 60 different oils are used and they can be taken by mouth, added to the bathwater, inhaled or used in massage oils. Although essential oils can be bought over the counter, it is advisable to consult a trained therapist before using them, as overdosing can be dangerous.

For more information contact the Aromatherapy Organizations Council, 3 Latymer Close, Braybrooke, Market Harborough, Leicester, LE16 8LN (01858 434242).

Bach flower remedies

These are simple essences of certain flowers, which are thought to transform the negative emotions to which people cling and which are expressed through physical illness. There are 38 different remedies used – the most well-known is probably the Bach Rescue Remedy – a good treatment for stress. Some NES members say they have benefited from this treatment.

For more information contact Dr Edward, Bach Centre, Mount Vernon, Sotwell, Wallingford, Oxon, OX10 0PZ (01491 834678).

Biochemical tissue salts

This is based on the theory that the body contains 12 essential mineral salts and that, if they get out of balance, illness results. The mineral salts which are lacking are then taken in minute forms to restore the balance. Tissue-salts are often prescribed by homeopaths but you can buy them yourself from health food shops (you should follow the guidelines for dosages on the container). The usual method is to dissolve them on your tongue without eating, drinking or cleaning your teeth for an hour afterwards. The following are particularly recommended:

- PMS and depression: Kali Phos
- heavy periods: Kali Phos, Silica
- fluid retention: Nat Mur or Nat Sulph
- painful periods: Mag Phos
- menstrual nausea: Combination S tissue salts.

Chinese medicine: see herbalism

Chiropractic

Like osteopathy (see below) chiropractic involves manipulating and adjusting the spine and other joints in the body. The basic idea is that the spine protects the spinal cord, and if it isn't aligned properly this can affect the nerve-supply, preventing the body from functioning properly, and resulting in illness. It is often used to treat back-pain and can be good for menstrual, bladder and constipation problems.

For more information contact the British Chiropractic Association, 29 Whitley Street, Reading, Berks. RG2 0EG (01734 757557).

Healing

No one quite knows how healing works, but with this technique, power is thought somehow to come through the healer's hands, helping to heal physical or emotional problems. Patients often say they experience feelings of cold or heat, or their skin tingling. There are different types of healing such as faith, spiritual and psychic healing.

For more information contact the National Federation of Spiritual Healers, Old Manor Farm Studio, Church Street, Sunbury on Thames, TW16 6RG (01932 783164); or the British Touch for Health Centre, 30 Suderly Road, Bognor Regis, PO21 1ER (01243 841689).

Herbalism

Herbs have been used for medicine throughout history and in every culture. The Chinese, Indians and native North Americans all have well-developed forms of herbal medicine – indeed, many of our own conventional medicines are derived from herbs.

Like other complementary therapists, the herbalist looks at the whole person, giving you a long initial consultation encompassing your life-style and medical history, and including routine blood-pressure and urine tests. Treatment is then prescribed in the form of syrups, tinctures (the alcoholic extract of a drug derived from a plant) or dried herbs to make up into an infusion of tea. Poultices, ointments and lotions may also be used externally.

Simple self-help remedies are available from health food shops or chemists. But for anything more serious you should consult a qualified herbalist who is trained to know exactly what herb to use, how to prepare and apply it, and how much to take.

For more information contact the National Institute of Medical Herbalists, 56 Longbrook Street, Exeter, Devon, EX4 6AH (01392 426022).

Endometriosis sufferers have found the following self-help herbal preparations useful:

For period pain and other twinges throughout the cycle: take one pinch of powdered ginger, or a few shreds of fresh root-ginger, infused in a cup of boiling water and sip at regular intervals. Honey can be used to sweeten the taste. Ginger works by relieving spasms and improving circulation. Pineapple juice can sometimes help: drink as much as you like during your period.

For bladder pain (when no infection is present): meadowsweet tea, which is made like ordinary tea and taken as a dose of one cupful (no milk) four times a day, or as required. A fresh batch should be made daily, although it can be reheated or kept in a thermos flask throughout the day.

For balancing hormones: Vitex Agnus Castus is recommended, but is best used under the supervision of herbalist. It is thought to affect the hormones produced by the pituitary gland, and is often recommended for menstrual problems as well as infertility. It should not be taken at the same time as hormone treatments.

Tummy problems: ginger, taken as an infusion, is good for wind problems and colicky pains. Slippery elm tablets can also be chewed (two before each meal) to counteract the irritant effects of some drugs on the stomach.

Chinese herbal remedies

Dong Quai: this helps with relaxation, and the pain and inflammation caused by PMS, pregnancy and the menopause. It has been used for thousands of years in China to nourish and strengthen the blood and regulate periods, and is thought to be particularly good at relieving period cramps.

White peony: in China, this is often used in combination with Dong Quai as a tonic for the nervous system. It also has a relaxing effect on the womb-muscles.

Leonuri: thought to invigorate the blood and help regulate periods. Helpful for irregular periods, premenstrual abdominal pain, infertility and water retention.

Black cohosh: from Native Americans, this may relieve painful or delayed menstruation, ovulation pain or period cramps. It is also thought to help balance female hormones.

For more information contact the Register of Chinese Herbal Medicine, RCHM, PO Box 400, Wembley, Middlesex HA9 9NZ (0181 904 1357).

Mexican yam

Mexican yam is a plant extract which contains diosgenin, the raw material from which progesterone can be made in a laboratory. It is thought to aid hormone balance and reduce stress, tiredness and menopausal symptoms (see Chapter 7 for more on the natural progesterone debate).

Homeopathy

There are five NHS homeopathic hospitals in Britain – in London, Glasgow, Liverpool, Bristol and Tunbridge – operating on an outpatient basis. To visit one you need to be referred by a GP or a medically-qualified homeopath. The Royal London Homeopathic Hospital in Great Ormond Street also runs a special women's clinic where they see a number of endometriosis sufferers.

Most patients are treated in the same way. First you are asked to fill in a detailed questionnaire about your whole life-style, including your mental state. You will then be prescribed a homeopathic remedy depending on the provoking situation, on what sort of pain you are experiencing and where you are feeling it. Remedies are made from natural substances such as minerals, herbs, salts, and even diseased tissues – all in microscopic dilutions. There are over 400 different remedies for abdominal pain alone, but common ones include thuja and sepia. Treatment can take anything from three months to a year. Some practitioners may also get a patient to write a diary of their emotional states and symptoms.

The main theory behind homeopathy is the idea that 'like cures like'. This means that the homeopath gives you minute amounts of whatever he thinks is causing the problem, and this is thought to stimulate your immune system into fighting the disease.

When taking homeopathic treatments you should avoid too much coffee and strongly-flavoured mints as they can interfere with the remedy's effect. Homeopaths can also offer natural remedies for the treatment of PMS and natural alternatives to HRT. Remedies can be taken alongside conventional drug-treatments, although you must inform the homeopath of any other drugs you are taking, because this could interfere with the treatment.

For a private therapist, contact: the British Homeopathic Association, 27a Devonshire Street, London W1N 1RJ (0171 935 2163).

Meditation

There are lots of different types of meditation, but all of them train your power of concentration to control your thoughts and calm your body. When meditating you are supposed to enter a trance-like state which, with practice, can lower your pulse and blood-pressure. It also reduces muscular tension and improves circulation. Local education authorities often hold classes, so you could look in the prospectus for a class near you. Alternatively you could go to a private teacher or centre which appeals to you. There are also plenty of good books around to teach you the basics of concentrating on your breathing and stilling your mind.

Maria says: 'I've been going to meditation at my local Buddhist centre for over a year and have found it has helped me reduce stress generally, as it helps me to take my everyday life at a much slower pace. It also helps with pain relief during my period. If I wake up in pain in the night, I concentrate on my breathing and before long I've found I've drifted off to sleep without even a painkiller!'

Osteopathy

This involves correcting structural defects of the spine in order to stimulate healing. For example, a misalignment of bones in the spine affects the nerves and blood-flow to other areas of the body, which if it continues, can cause disease. Treatment involves putting these defects right by stretching, massage and special exercises designed to relax the muscles and ligaments. It is thought to be particularly good for freeing blood from the pelvic area.

For more information contact the British Naturopathic & Osteopathic Association, 6 Netherall Gardens, London, NW3 5RR (0171 435 8728).

Reflexology

This is based on the idea that points on the feet are related to parts of the body. It involves massage and pressure applied to the feet either with the hands or a special vibrating device; this is then thought to provoke a reflex action in the corresponding organ or tissue. It is thought to be particularly good for menstrual problems, the menopause, headaches and high blood-pressure.

For more information contact the British Reflexology Association, Monks Orchard, Whitbourne, Worcester, WR6 5RB (01886 821207).

Shiatsu

This is based on the same principles as acupuncture, but instead of needles, the practitioner's own body is used to massage the areas where the energy flow is blocked. The practitioner may use anything from finger-and-thumb to elbow-and-knee pressure. This is supposed to release toxins and deep-seated tensions from the muscles, as well as stimulating the hormone system.

Sally says: 'I found that regular shiatsu sessions gave me space from pain and worry, and also gave me a good sense of my whole body.'

For more information contact the Shiatsu Society, 31 Pullman Lane, Godalming, Surrey, GU7 1XY (01483 860771).

Stress management

Some GPs' surgeries and hospitals run courses on how to cope with stress.

Eleanor attended a stress-management course: 'I learned deep-breathing exercises and took away some relaxation tapes on a stress management course run by my local surgery. I knew a lot of these techniques already, as I'm a nurse, but it still helped me to put them into practice. If you can just make a chink in the vicious circle of feeling in pain, then tired, then depressed and then in more pain, you can begin to reverse the effect.'

Visualization

Visualization has been found to help cancer sufferers, and is also considered a positive technique for endometriosis sufferers. It involves training your mind to think of positive pictures. Some exercises may also involve looking at the ways in which we may be unconsciously promoting endometriosis. For example, having endometriosis may be a roundabout way of reducing other people's demands on us, or of gaining rest because our life-style is too exhausting.

The NES (see Useful Addresses) produces a leaflet which gives a step-by-step guide to visualization to help endometriosis sufferers – an exercise which takes only about 15 minutes to do, and which could prove helpful.

Elizabeth, an endometriosis sufferer who benefited from acupuncture, also recommends the following books, which include visualization exercises which she has found helpful: *Love, Medicine and Miracles*, by Bernie Siegel; *How to Heal Your Life*, by Louise Hay; *Guided Meditations, Explorations and Healing*, by Stephen Levine (listed in Further Reading).

Elizabeth adds: 'I found some of the meditations, such as on how to soften the pain, moved me to tears. It was also a relief to see that someone else had also trodden the path I was travelling on. I also found the techniques useful in working with the pain instead of just taking painkillers.'

Yoga

Yoga is an oriental technique which involves learning particular postures, and breathing and relaxation exercises. It has been found to be especially helpful through its relaxing effects and because it can alter hormone production and restore the nervous system.

For more information contact the Yoga for Health Foundation, Ickwell Bury, Biggleswade, Bedfordshire, SG18 9EF (01767 627271).

How to choose a therapist

- *Ask your GP or someone you know to recommend a practitioner.*
- *Make sure they are a member of a recognized registered body with a code of practice (some of these are listed in Useful Addresses).*
- *Ask if they have treated anyone with endometriosis before.*
- *Look for someone you like and get on with.*
- *Ask how many treatments you might expect, the approximate cost and whether they offer a sliding scale of fees.*
- *Don't expect an instant cure – most alternative therapies are gentle and take a while to work.*

11

All Clear?

Is there a cure?

At the moment there is no cure for endometriosis; most of the treatments are about getting rid of the pain, restoring fertility and managing the illness generally. It is also not definitely known that endometriosis inevitably gets worse over time – if that were so, there would be more older women with more severe endometriosis. In fact, research suggests that endometriosis naturally resolves itself in 25 per cent of cases, and that in 50 per cent of cases it gradually moves from an active to a more passive form.

How often does it return?

Unfortunately none of the treatments are fool-proof. Hormonal treatments successfully treat pain in 85 per cent of cases, but it is not a permanent cure – and only 50 per cent of women with an endometrioma are helped by hormonal treatment, as the cysts tend to grow back afterwards. The exact recurrence rate of endometriosis after conservative surgery is not known – rates vary due to the lack of specific long-term studies. Recurrence rates after hysterectomy, if the ovaries remain, is 13 per cent within three years and 40 per cent after five years; in some cases, endometriosis returns even after the ovaries have been removed.

What to do when it comes back

If endometriosis does return, you may need to undergo a second treatment. But usually the recurrence must first be diagnosed to make sure it isn't something else causing the pain, such as post-surgical adhesions, pelvic inflammation or adenomyosis. As with the first treatment, your symptoms, the extent of the disease, your desire still to be able to have children, and any other complications, all have to be taken into account when deciding which treatment is best.

Learning to live with it

Emotionally a recurrence can be very difficult to handle. We often hang on to the belief that everything will be alright once it gets better. So you may feel you have failed in some way should endometriosis return. On top of that, you may have to deal with the feelings of others.

Jackie says: 'One difficulty can be the expectation of others. Friends, relations and colleagues are expecting the treatment to work, and initially they don't expect the endometriosis to return – so it becomes a process of all-round education.'

Coming to terms with the fact that you have a disease which may limit you in various ways, which could get better or worse, is difficult. You need to remind yourself that endometriosis isn't the whole of you, and that you can't just wait for a mythical future date when everything will be alright. You have to get on and make decisions in the here-and-now.

Everyone has different ways of doing this. Jackie has more useful advice on this subject:

'One thing I have learnt is persistence, and to glean all the information I can. As the endo society slogan goes, "Never give up" – and I won't.

Sometimes I visualize to myself a little cartoon entitled "Pain relief: shoot your doctor!" – which just helps during the frustrating times. I'm not an aggressive person – just more assertive!'

And if all else fails, remember that you are in good company. The following people have all managed to cope with endometriosis and lead fulfilling lives (and there are many more of us out there!): actress Marilyn Monroe; tennis player Mary Jo Fernandez; writer Hilary Mantel; Judith Church MP; actress Liza Goddard; TV presenter Jo Sheldon.

Your action plan

In a nutshell, this is what you should do:

1 Don't accept painful periods as normal.
2 Don't be embarrassed to discuss the symptoms.
3 Ask for explanations – again and again.
4 Keep a diary of events, detailing your pain, your periods and any associated problems.
5 Request a referral – you are allowed to ask for this.
6 If all else fails, consider changing your doctor or specialist. Contact your local CHC for advice on this.
7 Inform yourself. Gather as much information as you can from doctors

and nurses, from other sufferers, from self-help groups and from the NES.

Remember there *is* light at the end of the tunnel. And finally, good luck!

Useful Addresses

The two organizations specifically associated with endometriosis are:

National Endometriosis Society (NES)
Suite 50, Westminster Palace Gardens
1–7 Artillery Row, London SW1P 1RL
020-7222 2776
www.endo.org.uk   *0808 808 1257*
Send a large SAE for an info pack.

Irish Endometriosis Society
Carmichael House
North Brunswick Street, Dublin 7
Ireland
010 353 1873 5702

Other organizations which may be of help are listed below in alphabetical order.

Alcohol Concern
Waterbridge House
32–36 Loman Street, London SE1 0EE
020 7928 7377
www.alcoholconcern.org.uk

British Association of Counselling (BAC)
1 Regent Place
Rugby
Warwickshire CV21 2PJ
01788 562189
www.counselling.co.uk

British Association of Nutritional Therapists
BCM BANT
28 Old Gloucester Street,
London WC1N 3XX
0870 606 1284
www.bant.org.uk

CHILD
(Self-help for infertility)
Charter House
43 St Leonard's Road
Bexhill-on-Sea
East Sussex TN40 13A
01424 732361
www.child.org.uk

Council for Complementary and Alternative Medicine
206-208 Latimer Road
London W10 6RE
020-8968 3862

Council for Involuntary Tranquillizer Addiction
Cavendish House, Brighton Road
Waterloo
Liverpool L22 5NG
0151 474 9626
www.backtolife.uk.com

Eating Disorders Association
First Floor, Wensum House
103 Prince of Wales Road
Norwich NR3 1JE
01603 621414
www.eda.uk.com

Institute of Complementary Medicine
PO Box 194
London SE16 7QZ
020-7237 5165
www.icmedicine.co.uk

Institute of Optimum Nutrition
Blades Court
Deodar Road
Putney, London SW15 2NU
020-8877 9993
www.ion.ac.uk

ISSUE
(The National Fertility Association)
114 Lichfield Street
Walsall WS1 1SZ
01922 722888
www.issue.co.uk

National Association for Premenstrual Syndrome (NAPS`
2 East Point, High Street
Seal, Kent TN15 0EG
01732 459378
www.pms.org.uk

National Childbirth Trust (NCT)
Alexandra House, Oldham Terrace
London W3 6NH
08704 448707
www.nctpregnancyandbabycare.com

National Osteoporosis Society
Camerton, Bath BA2 0PJ
01761 471771

Nutrition Line (Higher Nature)
Burwash Common
East Sussex TN19 7LX
01435 882880

Pain Concern
PO Box 252
Crawley RH10 3GY
01293 552636
www.painconcern.fsnet.co.uk

RELATE (Marriage Guidance)
Herbert Gray College
Little Church Street
Rugby CV21 3AP
01788 573241
www.relate.org.uk

USEFUL ADDRESSES

SHE Trust
Red Hall Lodge Office
Red Hall Drive
Bracebridge Heath
Lincoln LN4 2JT
01522 519992
www.shetrust.org.uk
Email for free info pack at shetrust@bbheath.freeserve.co.uk

UNWIND
(Self-help for pain relief – run by correspondence only)
Melrose, 3 Alderley Close
Gilesgate
Durham DH1 1DS
0191 384 2056

Women's Environmental Network
PO Box 30626
London E1 1TZ
020-7481 9004
www.wen.org.uk

Women's Health
(Provides health information and also information about hysterectomy support groups)
52 Featherstone Street
London EC1Y 8RT
020-7251 6580

Women's Nutritional Advisory Service
(Supply women with an individually tailored diet for small fee)
PO Box 268
Lewes
East Sussex BN7 2QN
01273 487366
www.wnas.org.uk

Further Reading

General
Clark, Jan, *Hysterectomy and the Alternatives.* Virago, 1993.
Hay, Louise, *How to Heal Your Life.* Eden Grove.
Westcott, Patsy, *Alternative Healthcare for Women.* Grapevine/Thorsons, 1987.
Winn, Denise, *Well Woman Handbook.* Vermilion, 1995.

Chapter 7, Hysterectomy
Nicol, Rosemary, *Hormone Replacement Therapy: Your Guide to Making a Life Choice.* Vermilion, 1993.
Wilson, Dr Robert C. D., *Understanding HRT and the Menopause.* Which? Consumer Guides, 1995.

Chapter 8, Infertility
Brien, E. & Higgins, R., *Infertility – New Choices, New Dilemmas.* Penguin, 1995.
Winston, Prof. Robert, *Getting Pregnant.* Pan, 1993.

Chapter 9, Coping strategies
Carr, Allen, *The Easy Way to Stop Smoking.* Penguin, 1995.
Chaitow, Leon, *Candid Albicans: Could Yeast be your Problem?* Thorsons, 1995.
Kilmartin, Angela, *Candida – A Practical Handbook.* Bloomsbury Press, 1995.
Kingston, B. *Lifting the Curse.* Sheldon Press, 1982.
Maisner, Paulette with Turner, Rosemary, *The Food Trap: A Self-Help Guide to Control Your Eating Habits.* Allen & Unwin, 1985.
Quilliam, Susan & Grove-Stephenson, Ian, *The Counselling Handbook.* Thorsons.
Sadler, Jan, *Natural Pain Relief – A Practical Handbook of Self-Help.* Element Books, to be published early 1997.
Storch, M. & Carmichael, C., *Painless Periods.* Arlington Books, 1989.

Chapter 10, Complementary therapies
Levine, Stephen, *Guided Meditations, Explorations and Healing.* Gateway Books.
Siegel, Bernie, *Love, Medicine and Miracles.* Arran Books, 1989.

Index